Aromatherapy

For

Massage

Practitioners

Joy Burnett

License Notes

***

CONTENTS

Aromatherapy Is The Controlled Use Of Natural

Aromatic Oils, Which Are Obtained From Plants To

Achieve Balance And Harmony Of The Human Mind,

Body And Spirit.

AROMATHERAPY AS A TREATMENT

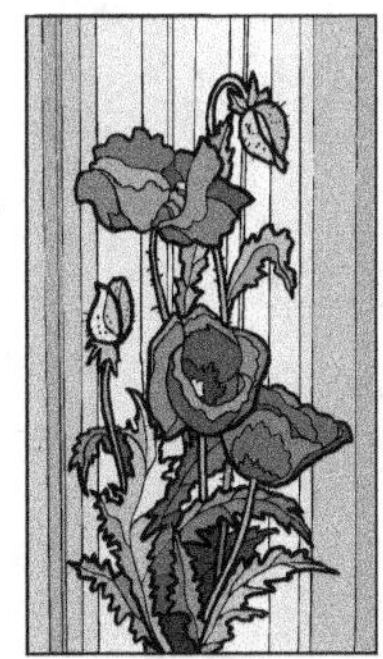

Any massage practitioner can enhance their treatments by using essential oils. Doing so offers a **non-toxic** treatment, which helps the **whole person**. With individually selected essential oils it can often alleviate symptoms and act as a natural trigger to help stimulate the body's own incredibly powerful healing ability. It can tip the balance between illness and good health.

In England, Aromatherapy is mainly known as a form of **beauty treatment** rather than as a **therapeutic discipline** and the possibilities have hardly been explored. Increased publicity and a need for alternative and complementary treatments have stimulated a growing interest in the subject. In traditional medicine, natural remedies have been used for centuries and because of growing concerns about the increasing use of strong synthetic drugs, medicine is turning once again toward nature's remedies.

Natural therapies generally speaking do not relieve instantly, which is what we have come to expect from our medicines. They are not magic potions but they assist the healing process, which is initiated in the hands–on massage or reflexology that you offer. Many of the oils do have powerful properties and each of these is fully explained in the individual description of the 40 oils in this book.

However a body that has been ravaged by tobacco, junk food, alcohol, anxiety, stress or overwork and neglect will not respond overnight to any kind of natural remedy.

True healing takes time and it has to be combined with a change in life style and attitude.

Aromatherapy can help many disorders, but for the best results it should form part of a ***Holistic*** health regime. We must look for the underlying causes of the presenting symptoms and treat as far as we can the whole person. As it is a natural therapy it aims to stimulate rather than suppress the body's natural defence mechanisms.

Nevertheless, it is possible to have quite a dramatic effect on some people. Those suffering with sinusitis, cramps, PMT and migraine, insomniacs and arthritics have often found these problems have been helped with a single treatment. Aromatherapy can be used in many ways.

A few suggestions are given later in this book.

HEALING TOUCH

Touch is one of the most basic forms of communication between people and often those who are not well, or are stressed, benefit simply by the touch of another human being. It is an extension of the instinctive urge to touch a painful or bruised part of the body. We automatically press certain points to relieve tension and stress-related pains and problems.

It is known that touch deprivation affects human happiness via the brain. Studies have shown that those individuals deprived of touch have a sparser, less developed branching structure in the cortex.

Giving and receiving 'touch' improves the immune functioning of the body. The elderly, children, and the terminally ill or anyone living with disease can benefit from the loving touch of someone who cares. Even a hug is a non-verbal way of communicating sympathy and love that we are not able to put easily into words.

Massage is a wonderful way to communicate and it can act as a preventative medicine – healing, soothing, and reassuring.

Confidence in the area of touch does not come easily to some people – in fact, many children have been brought up without being adequately touched or fondled and this can result in a lifetime of craving affection and the need to be 'babied'.

This brings us to appropriate and non-appropriate touch.

Touch has become confused with sex: man / woman / homosexuality / child abuse etc. We have very few culturally condoned ways of expressing friendships through touch.

Touch is about trust and feeling safe. It is the ultimate in non-verbal communication. It is healing and we all have healing powers. Massage provides the means for patient – healer contact. Our hands are very sensitive and can discover things in the body that tell us a great deal about the person with whom we are dealing. They can feel congestion, tension, swelling, skin texture and sensitivities.

Between practitioner and patient it must always be a symbiotic relationship, the hands transmitting energy and receiving information at the same time.

Semyon Kirlian discovered that all living things have an 'aura' of energy that can be photographed with a special technique. The Kirlian experiments show quite clearly that energy can be increased when the healer is mentally focused on healing. The fact that we can control energy by our thought processes suggests that we all have the ability to heal.

In order to heal you must be able to feel – feel sympathy, compassion and care for the person you are treating. Therefore, the more concentrated thought you put into a massage, the more the flow of healing energy will be transmitted.

Some forms of massage aim only to benefit the physical body by easing tense or tight muscles or increasing circulation but even so a general feeling of well being will usually result. The benefits of massage are cumulative and a regular massage will prolong the feelings of well being forever increasing periods, after each treatment.

By using plant oils that have been carefully chosen, the massage becomes a therapeutic treatment. As you will see, the oils influence on several different levels, the physical, emotional and spiritual. Although we may perceive these levels as separate, they are in fact interrelated. There are many different ways to use essential oils but massage is by far the most important application of Aromatherapy.

As you study the oils, you will become aware of the many and different individual qualities they have, and how they can be used to create specific effects. An ***Individual Prescription*** will help the body's natural ability to heal itself. It can trigger responses in the body that help protect it from virus and bacteria and relieve problems (and without side effects).

Different practitioners have quite different ways of giving massage, depending on their training and background and also partly on their personal outlook and preferences. There are a variety of techniques and providing a therapist has been thoroughly trained and uses it with care and a nurturing attitude towards the person who needs help, it doesn't matter too much which method is used.

What is most important is that the technique used is flowing and the order of the movements in your massage should direct the flow of lymphatic fluid around the body. Develop your style and rhythm as you go.

WHAT ARE ESSENTIAL OILS?

Essential oils are liquid mixtures of compounds obtained from plants. They are the natural *odorific constituents* of the plant. They are not really oils at all but complicated cocktails of many different *chemicals* such as *esters, terpenes, oxides, phenols, lactones,* and *aldehydes.* They are usually secreted from *glands, ducts,* or *cells* in one or several parts of the aromatic plants.

They should not feel greasy, and although the consistency and colours of essential oils vary, they should feel fluid and non-oily. When buying essential oils, make sure that they have the Latin name on the label so that you can identify the different chemo-types. Although there are many synthetic copies and products that are mixed ready for massage, only the pure natural oil is therapeutic on a health level.

It takes a great deal of work to produce a tiny amount of essential oil; 6 million *Rose* blossoms are required to produce 1 ounce of rose oil and 8 million hand picked *Jasmine* blossom to produce one kilo of Jasmine oil. It becomes obvious why Jasmine is one of the most expensive oils on the market.

Because the essential oils are so sweet smelling it might be easy to suppose that their value is essentially one of charm. Not true! These substances are very complex in their molecular structure and very effective.

The essential oil of **Oregano** for example is 26 times more powerful as an antiseptic than phenol – which is the active ingredient in many commercial cleaning materials and **Tea Tree** oil is 11-12 times more antiseptic than carbolic acid or phenol, so it is effective against a range of bacterial, viral and fungal conditions.

So, essential oils are not manufactured and they are not necessarily harmless.

The strength at which the essential oil is used is very important, because some, if used in excess, or applied too strong, have the reverse effect to that which is desired.

For example a low concentrate of **Peppermint** oil applied to an itchy skin will relieve the irritation. A strong concentration will aggravate the condition. Similarly **Digitalis**, which is the essential oil of foxglove, is poisonous in high concentrates, but used carefully in medicine, it is very effective in relieving heart conditions. Digitalis is not used in Aromatherapy treatments.

It is important that the correct **quantity** and the correct **concentration** are used, as it does not follow that the more we use the better will be the result.

See ***PROPORTIONS***

Because the aromatic molecules of the essential oils are tiny fat-soluble substances they are easily absorbed through the skin during a massage or when applied locally. Once they pass through the cutaneous surface, they make their way to the dermis. The molecules enter the general circulation via the capillaries there. They can have a profound effect both on the physical, emotional, and general health.

The pleasure of aromas cannot be denied and they affect us on many levels, sometime deep within our subconscious mind. They can have a profound impact on our physiological and psychological wellbeing. That is why it is important to mix an aromatherapy product with the ***individual*** in mind. It is not intended to take the place of ***conventional*** medicine and should not be used to treat serious medical or psychological problems.

There are many and varied uses for natural essential oils and they are indispensable to medicine, to food / drink, where they are used as flavour-enhancers and food preservatives and in the cosmetic industries. Manufacturers of beauty products appreciate their cell rejuvenating and healing properties, while the fragrance industry is more concerned with their delightful aromas and their mood and emotion enhancing capacities.

Many oils are active ingredients in commonly used drugs or are an inspiration for chemical copies.

Essential oils are volatile and completely different from the base oils (***Almond, Grapeseed, Jojoba, etc***) that we use to apply the essential oils to the body. The base massage oils are also called fixed oils and do not evaporate as essential oils do.

Essential oils are obtained from different parts of the plant:
Leaves (***Eucalyptus***) – Wood (***Sandalwood***) – Bark (***Cinnamon***) – Flowers (***Rose***) – Roots (***Carrot***) – Rhizomes *(**Ginger**)* – Berries (***Juniper***) – Seeds (***Fennel***) – Fruits (***Lemon***)

Specific oils are obtained from different parts of the same plant:
From the Bitter Orange Tree (Seville or Bigarade) – Citrus aurantium, 3 different oils are extracted

Neroli oil is derived from the blossom of the tree. ***Petitgrain*** comes from the leaf. ***Orange*** comes from the fruit.

Clove Oil – Eugenia Caryophyllata. Clove oil comes from the leaves and stem. ***Clove bud*** oil from the buds only.

There are a few oils that are extracted from grasses such as ***Palmarosa, and Lemongrass and Vetiver.***

It is important to consider the high rate of evaporation and the affect on the person being treated when combining a well-balanced mixture. The volatility rate varies in different oils and most essences fall into one of the following three classifications:

TOP NOTES – The smallest molecules are the fastest acting, the quickest to evaporate, the most stimulating and uplifting to mind and body.

They contain mostly highly volatile, small molecules and the aroma will therefore last only about 24 hours.

MIDDLE NOTES – Mixed sized molecules, moderately volatile, primarily affects the functions of the body. Balancing oils. These contain a mixture of high and low volatile molecules and will last 2 to 4 days.

BASE NOTES – Heavier molecules, slower to evaporate. Sedative and relaxing. It is worth noting that a mixture of top note with base note will hold back the volatility of the top note. Being mostly low volatile molecules the aroma can last up to 6 days.

You can check the volatility of your oils by putting a drop on paper and smelling at regular intervals. You will soon see that the top note last the least amount of time. The distinctive strength of Holistic aromatherapy as a healing art depends upon:

- *The chemical components of the essential oils.*
- *The base / fixed oil used.*
- *The hands-on skills of the practitioner. The massage or reflexology treatment*
- *The time taken to blend an individual prescription.*
- *The problems / condition / age of the client*
- *Olfaction*

SAFETY AND PRECAUTIONS

Before embarking on using the essential oils in treatments for yourself or others, it is wise to study the oil profiles carefully. Aromatherapy oils should always be treated with respect. They will serve you well if you observe a few basic rules.

1. Never use undiluted oils directly on the skin. One or two of the oils can be used neat in certain circumstances but do not be tempted unless you know exactly what you are doing.

2. Dilute your oils with water, carrier oil, lotion, milk or hydrosol (floral water).

3. Avoid contact with eyes. Wash with carrier oil, milk or water if any oils get in the eyes.

4. Avoid exposing skin treated with oils to sunlight, especially the citrus oils, **Lemon, Bergamot, Orange, Grapefruit and Mandarin.**

5. Certain oils should not be used if homeopathic remedies are being taken, Particularly **Eucalyptus, Basil and Peppermint**, which can neutralise the effect of the remedy.

6. Essential oils that are not stored well, do go off and can cause an allergic reaction.

7. Ingestion of essential oils is not recommended.

8. Observe the rules that apply during pregnancy.

9. Do not use cheap or adulterated oils.

10. Stick to recommended doses.

11.   Oils are highly inflammable so keep away from naked flames or excess heat.

12.   Label and date all oils carefully and precisely.

13.   Essential oils that should only be used by a qualified Aromatherapist and considered unsafe for home use include: **Aniseed, Origanum, Thyme Savory, Caraway, Clove, Tagetes, Tarragon, Sage, Hyssop, Camphor, Cinnamon, Wintergreen.**

14.   Always store essential oils out of the reach of children and pets.

PROPORTIONS

Proportions are important and the following is a guideline only:

Preparing Massage Oil or Lotion for the Body

A general guideline for the amount of base oil is the patients dress size for ladies (size 12 = 12mls) and the chest measurement halved for men (40ins halved 20ins = 20mls)

The *Treatment oil* referred to is the total number of drops of essential oil added to the carrier or base oil and the larger number is the *Maximum* amount to be used. It may be made up of drops from 2-4 different essential oils.

When using a mixture of essential oils as *Treatment oil* it is a good idea to put them together in one bottle or jar. With this method you can then make massage oils or lotions easily and economically and also have some treatment oil left over for a bath, for inhaling, or to use in the next bottle of carrier oil or lotion.

To 50 mls Carrier oil or lotion: 15-25 drops of *Treatment* oil.

To 100 mls of Carrier oil or lotion: add 30-50 drops of *Treatment* oil

To 200 mls of Carrier oil or lotion: add 60-100 drops of *Treatment* oil.

Typical Massage Strengths:

12 mls carrier oil.   Maximum 6 drops essential oil.

20mls carrier oil.   Maximum 10 drops essential oil.

10 ml cream   1-2 drops essential oil.

DOSES SHOULD BE HALVED FOR THE ELDERLY AND YOUNG CHILDREN.

EXTRACTION PROCESSES

Some plant material, especially those with delicate flowers deteriorate very quickly after harvesting so have to be extracted 'on the spot' The method of extraction depends on the quality and delicacy of the plant material and the type of end product that is required.

Steam Distillation – This is a process that consists of placing plant material in a container called a 'still', together with water. The water is brought to the boil and as the plants are heated the essential oils are extracted along with other substances from the plant material, together with the steam from the water. It is passed into an outlet at the top of the still which carries the mixture of steam and oil vapour to the condenser, a cooling coil which is immersed in cold water whereby the steam condenses back to water and essential oil content condenses back to essential oil.

The oil and water quickly separate due to the difference in specific gravity and the essential oil floats on the top of the water. It is therefore easily collected. The high temperatures can be harmful to some of the more fragile ingredients and the whole process requires delicate handling and expertise. Distillation time varies but in general the time taken is between 45 minutes and 2 hours. The water used in the process should be obtained from a spring if possible because it produces a good quality essential oil. The choice of material of which the still is made is also important, and modern stills are usually made of stainless steel.

Expression – This method is used mainly to release oil from the skin of citrus fruits. The outer peel of the fruits is mechanically pressed and the liquid is absorbed into sponges attached to wooden blocks. The sponges are then squeezed, and the resultant oil collected and filtered. This process is used for bergamots, lemons, limes, oranges, and mandarin.

Maceration – This is a process whereby the plant oils are extracted by soaking the plant material in a warmed base or fixed oil. This produces scented oil that can be used for massage

Extraction processes are important to understand as they dictate the end product, whether essentials or absolutes.

Other processes used are ***Solvent Extraction, Cold Process Enfleurage*** and ***Hydro-diffusion.***

THE MANY USES OF ESSENTIAL OILS

Inhalation

This is probably the quickest way into the blood stream by the interchange of gases in the lungs. The lungs are lined with a rich blood supply, which readily absorbs the essential oil molecules. These then travel around the body for several hours before they are eliminated. The tiny molecules also enter directly into the nervous system via the Olfactory Nerve.

The Olfactory centre is very closely linked with the limbic system in the brain, which is the seat of our emotions and feelings. This extremely active system is connected to other vital parts of the brain involved in controlling heart rate, blood pressure, breathing, memory, and reaction to stress. Therefore smells can evoke pleasant or unpleasant responses and memories.

Certain oils stimulate specific neuro-chemicals within the nervous system.

It is worth remembering that is necessary for the recipient to like the aroma of the oils being used.

The smell of the oils can affect the mood and general well being and as every single human being is different. That is why a ***specialised individual prescription*** is required.

For quick inhalation, 2-4 drops of your chosen oil can be added to hot water, put into a vaporiser, or added to a professional steamer.

Add 2 drops to hot water placed in a bowl. Drape a towel over the head and bowl and inhale. This method should not to be used by children, asthmatics or by people with poor or weak veins on their face.

Absorption – Whole Body Massage

Massaged into the skin, where the touch of masseur's hands also plays a part. The oils enter the lymph and blood stream through the skin by diffusion (the volatile oil turns into a gas in liquid form and enters the body via the sweat, oil glands and hair follicles). Large amounts of subcutaneous fat will impede absorption as will water retention and poor circulation. It activates the nerve endings and stimulates the circulation of the blood and lymph.

The massage itself is usually simple *Effleurage, Petrissage and Friction* sometimes combined with the use of pressure points. It should be relaxing and restoring. The benefits are often not felt until the following day and sometimes several treatments are necessary if the patient is particularly tense or in pain. The benefit of massage is usually cumulative and can be used as a preventative medicine as well as a curative one.

Specific problem areas: For bad backs, arthritic joints, strained muscle pain, stomach disorders, sinus pain and headaches or any problem where oil is going to be used on specific areas slightly more essential oil can be used, i.e. 6-9 drops to 12 mls base oil if it is only going to be applied to a small area of the body.

Bathing: Use only the gentle oils. Add 4-10 drops to your bath after the water is run or dilute with a little vegetable oil or milk if your skin is dry. Lie for 10-15 minutes.

Sitz or Bidet: To aid healing after childbirth and for helping with genital or anal infections. 2-3 drops. Sit or bathe for 10-15 minutes.

Footbath: Lovely for tired aching feet, fungal or skin problems on the feet. A nice way to give the benefits of essential oils to the elderly and infirm. 2-3 drops, soak for 10-15 minutes.

Compress: For painful joints, shoulder or back pain. Dilute with carrier oil as for massage. Apply and cover.

For swelling and inflammation, soak a soft cloth and cool in the freezer, then add a couple of drops of your chosen oil to the cloth, and apply to the affected area.

If warmth is necessary, dilute your oils in warm water and then soak a soft cloth in the water and apply to the affected area.

Facial Lotion, Cream, and Gels: Specific skin problems like acne and spots. General skin care. 10 mls cream or lotion to 1-2 drops of essential oil.

Jacuzzi: 3 drops per person to keep bacteria away.

Sauna: 2 drops per 600mls of water. Mix with water beforehand and throw it on the heat source as normal. Use only **Eucalyptus, Tea Tree, or Pine**. Bear in mind that the body will not absorb the oil whilst perspiring but the inhalation will be beneficial.

Apply your diluted oils to your body after it has cooled down.

Other Ideas

Perfume bed linen, notepaper, clothes, or carpets with a few drops of oil. Can also be used on pillows and handkerchiefs, light bulbs and as a room freshener. Add a few drops of your favourite oil to the last rinse when washing your hair. **Chamomile** for blondes and **Rosemary** for brunettes.

Many of our Essential oils can be used in cooking. Add **Orange, Lemon,** or **Peppermint** to your desserts, cakes or biscuits, and a drop of one of the herbal or citrus oils in oil and vinegar to create a wonderful salad dressing.

In the garden, some of the oils are very effective against aphids and greenfly. Try **Basil, Thyme, Lavendin, Lavender, Peppermint,** or **Cedarwood** diluted (about 8 drops to a small bucket of water). Can be sprayed onto rose bushes.

Note: Some Essential Oils will stain delicate materials.

ESSENTIAL OIL HOUSEKEEPING

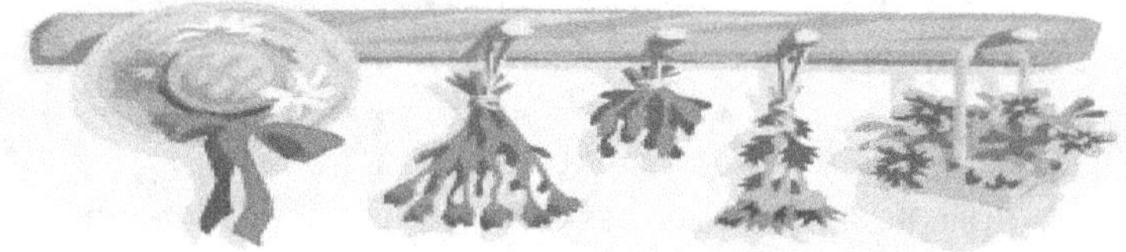

As you can see there are many ways of using Essential oils besides massage. If you have a stock of oils one of the ways you can enhance your life is by using them for cleaning and refreshing your home.

All essential oils are highly antiseptic although some are more so than others. Many oils are more powerful as an antiseptic than phenol, a common antiseptic chemical used in many cleaning products.

Many essential oils have anti-fungal properties so are useful for areas where food is stored. The anti-bacterial properties of oils like **Lavender, Lemon, Ravensara, Sweet Marjoram, Tea Tree and Lemongrass** make them ideal for cleaning areas like worktops, waste bins and pet beds.

Being natural chemicals they will not contaminate the waterways into which so much of our daily waste is routinely deposited. The tiny quantities required means they are safe and also make them highly economical.

There is a great deal of research being done into the value of these lovely products and we know that good quality oils used properly can make sure that your home is germ and bacteria free, fragrant and clean.

A few ideas:

Fridge cleaning, Worktops, Floors: 1 drop of **Lemon or Geranium** and 1 drop of **Grapefruit** in 1 pint of water.

Waste bins: Add 2 drops of **Tea Tree, Lavender or Lemongrass** to a damp cloth.

Pet Care: Clean plastic and wicker baskets with a damp cloth onto which you have added 2 drops of Lemon, **Lavender, Cedarwood or Tea Tree**. When washing their bedding add 4 drops of oil to the final rinse cycle. For keeping pets clean and free from tics and fleas, sprinkle a few drops of **Juniper, Cedarwood, Lavender, or Tea Tree** on their bedding or use 4-5 drops in their bath water. Mixed with water or alcohol the oils can be rubbed into or brushed through your pet's coat.

Airing cupboard: Fold a tissue or a cotton wool pad and add 4 drops of **Cedarwood, Lavender, Geranium, Sandalwood, Patchouli or Ylang Ylang**. Base notes obviously last the longest. This can be placed between towels, sheets and duvet covers. Make a blend you really like and use in all your drawers and cupboards. Incidentally most of these oils are moths and insect repellents too.

Fresh Air Spray: Mix 10 drops of your favourite oil or blend and add to 100 mls of water pump action spray and you have a chemical free way of making your home smell fragrant as well as keeping it germ free.

Smelly footwear: Put 2-3 drops of **Lemongrass, May Chang or Lavender** onto an unused dry teabag. Leave in the offending footwear.

GLOSSARY OF TERMS USED
TO DESCRIBE ESSENTIAL OILS

This list that follows aims to show some of the most important properties and uses of the oils. It is by no means exhaustive.

ANALGESIC	Relieves pain
ANTIFUNGAL	Prevents fungal infection
ANAPHRODISIAC	Decreasing sexual desire
ANTICONVULSIVE	Prevents convulsions
ANTIDEPRESSANT	Alleviates depression
ANTIDIABETIC	Improves circulatory problems
ANTI-INFLAMMATORY	Reduces inflammation
ANTISEPTIC	Inhibits the growth of bacteria
ANTISPASMODIC	Relieves spasm especially in smooth muscle
ANTISUDORIFIC	Reduces perspiration
ANTIVIRAL	Inhibits viral infection
APHRODISIAC	Increases sexual desire
BACTERICIDAL	Inhibits bacterial infection
BECHIC	Reduces or relieves coughing
CARMINATIVE	Eases colic and flatulence
CEPHALIC	Mental stimulants for poor concentration

CHOLAGOGIC	Stimulates the flow of bile to the intestines
CICATRISANT	Promoting healing and the formation of scar tissue
CORDIAL	A tonic for the heart
CYTOPHYLACTIC	Stimulating the production of new cells
DECONGESTANT	Helps diminish catarrhal blockage
DEPURATIVE	Blood cleansing
DETOXIFYING	Helps cleanse body of impurities
DIURETIC	Stimulates the secretion of urine
EMMANOGOGIC	Hormonal balancing
EXPECTORANT	Helps removal of phlegm and catarrh
FEBRIFUGE	Helps reduce fever
GALACTOGOGIC	Increases secretion of breast milk
HAEMOSTATIC	Stops bleeding
HEPATIC	A tonic for the liver
HYPERTENSIVE	Raises blood pressure
HYPOTENSIVE	Lowers blood pressure
INSECTICIDE	Insect repellent
IMMUNOSTIMULANT	Supports the immune system
NERVINE	A nerve tonic

PARTURIENT	Aids childbirth
RUBERFACIENT	Warming. Stimulates circulation locally
SEDATIVE	Calming. Inducing sleep
STIMULANT	Increasing activity and wakefulness
STOMACHIC	Tonifies the stomach
TONIC	Invigorating
UTERINE	Giving tone to the uterus
VASODILATOR	Causes small blood vessels to expand
VASDOCONSTRICTOR	Causes constriction of the blood vessels
VERMIFUGE	Eliminates intestinal worms
VULNERARY	Helps healing of wounds

34

STUDY OF 40 ESSENTIAL OILS

1. BASIL – OCIMUM BASILICUM

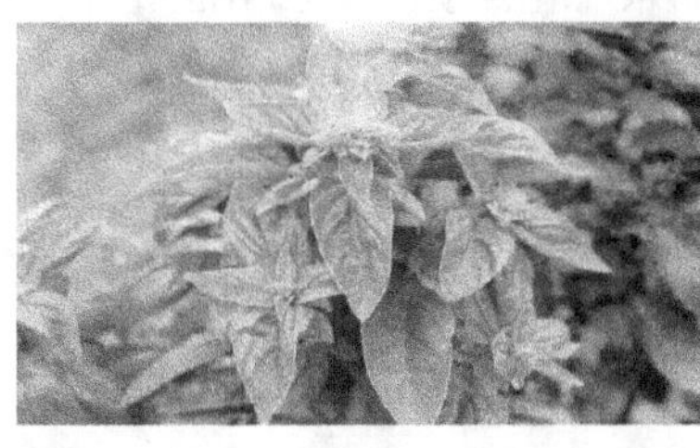

Steam distilled from the flowering tops and young shoots of the plant. The oil is a pale yellow with an aromatic, warm, clean aroma. Originally from India and North Africa it is now cultivated throughout Europe, The Pacific Islands, North and South America.

PROPERTIES: Analgesic, Antidepressant, Antiseptic, Antispasmodic, Aphrodisiac, Carminative, Cephalic, Digestive, Emmenagogic, Expectorant, Febrifuge, Galactagogic, Insecticide, Nervine, Stomachic, Sudorific, Tonic, and Vermifuge.

USES: A good tonic for the nervous system and is useful for clearing the head and mental fatigue. It sharpens the senses and encourages concentration.

Because of its Cephalic properties it is good for headaches, migraine, nasal and ear congestion. It is cleansing and is therefore useful for any problems of congestion of the Respiratory or Digestive systems.

In Ayurvedic and Chinese medicine it is used for many digestive disorders. It helps cleanse the kidneys and improves the blood circulation.

Considered 'cooling'. It is good for inflamed conditions, rheumatism, fevers etc.

Has a refreshing and tonic action on the skin and once again is good for congested skin problems. It is said to imitate the oestrogen hormone and is useful for menopausal problems and such things as scanty periods, lack of ovulation and tender breasts.

TOP NOTE WHICH BLENDS WELL WITH: Geranium, Bergamot, Clary sage, Rosemary, Lavender and Hyssop.

CAUTIONS: There are many varieties of this plant and the chemical constituents vary considerably. It is important to only use oils with a low content of Methyl chavicol as this is moderately toxic and recent studies suggest that in large doses it could cause cancer. To be avoided during pregnancy but helpful during labour.

2. BENZOIN – STYRAX BENZOIN

Usually Solvent extracted from the gum resin of the tree, which is produced by cutting the tree bark. The gum is collected after it hardens. It is treacle-like oil and it is brownish / red. It has a strong aroma of sweet vanilla. It is grown in Java, Sumatra and Thailand, Laos, China and Vietnam. It is an ABSOLUTE.

PROPERTIES: Anti-inflammatory, Anti-catarrhal, Antiseptic, Astringent, Carminative, Cicatrisant, Cordial, Deodorant, Diuretic, Expectorant, Sedative, and Vulnerary.

USES: It is best known in the form of compound tincture of Benzoin, or Friars balsam. It is another of the long known oils and has been used in different forms for centuries.

Primitive Malays used Benzoin in the form of ointment and fumigation for medicinal and ceremonial purposes.

The Chinese use it for its antiseptic qualities and urinary infections such as cystitis and urethritis.

It is extremely penetrating and is used for painful rheumatism or arthritis.

A few drops added to the final hair rinse will help scalp conditions. It is especially useful for psoriasis, eczema, and other skin conditions such as bedsores, ulcers, and burns.

All respond well to Benzoin.

Grounding and warming, calming and reassuring in times of mental or physical upheaval or stress.

Mixed with Eucalyptus it is excellent for catarrh and chest infections, bronchitis, and asthma. Inhalation is recommended.

Mixed with Lemon it is an ideal skin toner. Because of its dense sweet aroma it mixes well with the sharper aromas.

BASE NOTE WHICH BLENDS WELL WITH: Lemon, Eucalyptus, Sandalwood, Rose, and Frankincense.

CAUTIONS: Possibility of skin reaction in sensitive people.

3. BERGAMOT – CITRUS BERGAMIA

Expressed from the peel of the nearly ripe fruit, the oil is a pale greenish / yellow changing to a deeper colour as it ages. It has a fruity, slightly spicy aroma, which is a mixture of orange and lemon. It is grown in Italy and it is said to have been exported by Christopher Columbus from the Canary Islands. Not to be confused with Herb Bergamot or Bee balm (Monarda didyma).

PROPERTIES: Analgesic, Anti-depressant, Antiseptic, Antispasmodic, Carminative, Cicatrisant, Expectorant, Diuretic, Febrifuge, Laxative, Rubifacient, Stimulant, Stomachic, Tonic, Vermifuge, and Vulnerary.

USES: Antispasmodic on the digestive system and is therefore useful for colic and indigestion.

Said to help encourage poor appetites so it could be useful for helping those suffering with Anorexia. Calming to the respiratory system and helps bronchitis and sore throats.

For the Genito-Urinary system it is excellent as it can calm the symptoms of thrush, cystitis, leucorrhoea, and puritis. A wonderful oil for treating cold sores and several other skin conditions such as eczema, psoriasis, wounds, shingles, scabies, chicken pox, varicose ulcers and acne. It is calming for the nervous system so is useful for agitation and insomnia. It is helpful for problems of lethargy caused by stressful situations as it has uplifting as well as calming properties.

It is used extensively in the food and beverage industries, notably in Earl Grey tea. It is the ingredient of many perfumes and Eau de Colognes.

TOP NOTE, WHICH BLENDS WELL WITH: Lavender, Neroli, Jasmine, Juniper, Geranium, Chamomile, Patchouli and Ylang Ylang.

CAUTIONS: A non-toxic oil but care should be taken as Bergaptene is phototoxic and exposure to sunlight can cause a reaction and discoloration of the skin. Particular care is needed with very fair skins or large moles. Bergaptene free oil is available to Aromatherapists if they are happier to use it but remember it is not complete

4. BLACK PEPPER – PIPER NIGRUM

One of the oldest-known spices. It is steam distilled from the crushed, dried fruit of the plant. The oil is a pale yellow mobile liquid with a sharp, fresh spicy smell. It is cultivated in the East mainly Singapore, India, China, Madagascar and Malaysia. It is also often distilled in the USA.

PROPERTIES: Analgesic, Antiseptic, Anti-spasmodic, Aphrodisiac, Cardiac, Carminative, Detoxifying, Digestive, Diuretic, Febrifuge, Laxative, Rubifacient, Stimulant, Stomachic, Tonic.

USES: It stimulates the digestive tract; therefore it is good for constipation, and congestion. It promotes urine and stimulates the kidneys.

Aids the digestion of protein and generally expels toxins.

It has been suggested that it is a possible antidote for fish and mushroom poisoning.

It is a circulatory stimulant and is a excellent warming oil for the muscles both before and after strenuous exercise.

Very helpful for aches, pains or overtiredness and is particularly good for sciatica, rheumatism, and arthritis.

Mixed with Geranium, use for chilblains.

It is said to aid the formation of new blood cells so it may be useful for anaemia.

Helps reduce cellulite and treats bruises.

Its stimulant effect on the nervous systems makes it useful oil for treating lethargy.

MIDDLE NOTE, WHICH BLENDS WELL WITH: All the flower and citrus oils, Frankincense, Sandalwood, and Vetivert.

CAUTIONS: The undiluted oil can irritate the skin. Always dilute well.

Overuse could damage the kidneys.

Do not use on highly nervous people.

5. CEDARWOOD – CEDRUS ATLANTICA

Distilled from the wood of the tree. It is a yellow to deep amber, viscous oil with an aroma that is warm and woody with a hint of balsam and turpentine. Native to the Atlas Mountains of Algeria the oil is mainly produced in Morocco.

There are other species of Cedarwood and the oldest recorded is Cedrus Libani from Lebanon. This was most probably the oil used by the Ancient Egyptians for embalming, building and shipbuilding. Although closely related to Cedrus Atlantica, it is scarce due to over use.

PROPERTIES: Antiseptic, Aphrodisiac, Astringent, Diuretic, Expectorant, Fungicide, Insecticide, Sedative, and Tonic.

USES: Its astringent qualities make it ideal for acne, fungal infections, greasy skin, dandruff and hair loss. Cold and chest infections respond well to this oil. It has the ability to break down mucus so it helps with the treatment of catarrhal conditions especially chronic bronchitis.

It is a useful oil for problems of the Genito-Urinary system and particularly helpful with Cystitis. Good for general aches and pains.

Mixed with Rose or Lavender it has a sedative effect and is good for anxiety and tension.

It has a tonic and cleansing effect on the kidneys and lymph.

Considered to be a sexual stimulant, it is used extensively in masculine perfumes and aftershave. It is also a useful insect repellent.

BASE NOTE, WHICH BLENDS WELL WITH: Rose, Lavender, Juniper, Patchouli, and Benzoin.

CAUTIONS: Do not use Cedarwood produced in the U.S.A, they are a different species and have different properties. These oils are used mainly in the perfume industries and are not suitable for therapeutic purposes. Cedarwood is a good substitute for the more expensive Sandalwood.

6. CHAMOMILE GERMAN – MATRICARIA CHAMOMILIA

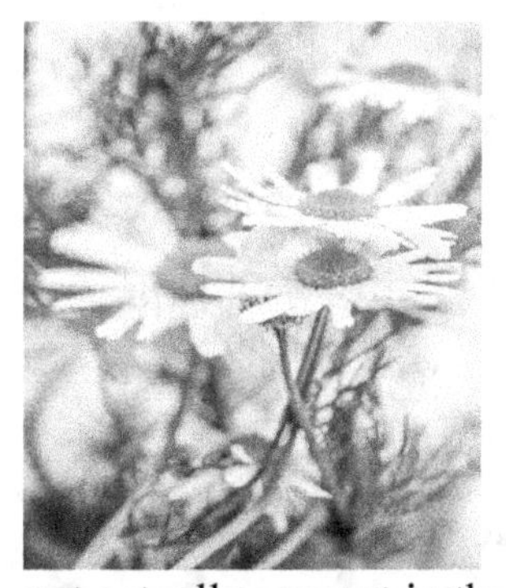 Steam distilled from the flowers of the plant, the oil varies from pastel blue / green to dark greenish / blue.

The oil from Matricaria Chamomilia is usually very dark in colour because of its high Azulene content. Azulene is a powerful anti-inflammatory agent that is not actually present in the plant but is formed in the production of the oil.

Therefore Matricaria Chamomilia is a more potent remedy for inflammatory conditions than Anthemis Nobilis. It has a refreshing earthy aroma and was at one time cultivated in Germany, hence its name.

There is another Chamomile available; *Ormenis Mixta or Moroccan Chamomile* which, possess similar properties to the true chamomile but it belongs to a different botanical family.

USES: Invaluable for skin conditions such as eczema, urticaria and dry / flaky conditions. As skin problems are often related to stress responses Chamomile is invaluable as both a Sedative and Anti-inflammatory treatment.

Use in cold compresses for swellings. It has been used successfully on burns, inflamed ulcers and boils. As it is Carminative, it soothes the stomach relieving gastritis, diarrhoea, colitis, nausea and may be helpful when treating Irritable Bowel Syndrome.

Good for female disorders, including scanty menstruation, painful or irregular periods, and excessive loss of blood during long periods and menopausal problems. Its action on the liver makes it useful for treating jaundice.

On a psychological level, Chamomile is good for anger and heated emotions. It is often useful to use when insomnia is due to anxiety, over excitement or excessive worry. Being so gentle it can safely be used on children and the elderly.

MIDDLE NOTE, WHICH BLENDS WELL WITH: Benzoin, Bergamot, Geranium, Lavender, Lemon, Neroli, Rose, Patchouli and Ylang Ylang.

CAUTIONS: Should be avoided during the early months of pregnancy.

7. CLARY SAGE – SALVIA SCLAREA

Steam distilled from the flowering tops of the plant plus leaves and stalks. The oil is clear to pale yellow green and it has a warm, sweet nutty odour. It is native to Southern Europe but it is cultivated worldwide. The best oils are produced in France and Hungary.

Sometimes called 'eyebright' because water distilled from the leaves and flowers can be used to bathe the eyes to clear away soreness and give them a sparkle. *Sclarea – latin for clear.* It was introduced into England in the 16th century.

PROPERTIES: Antidepressant, Antiseptic, Antispasmodic, Aphrodisiac, Carminative, Deodorant, Emmenagogic, Hypotensive, Nervine, Parturient, Sedative, Stomachic, and Tonic.

USES: It is strongly antispasmodic so it is useful in any condition that needs calming such as pre-menstrual cramps, inflamed skin conditions or digestive problems.

It also helps relieve asthma as it relaxes the bronchial tubes. It is a powerful muscle relaxant so it is especially useful where muscular tension arises from mental or emotional states.

It is often used in the last stage of labour to improve the efficiency of uterine contractions. It is said that it can induce dramatic and colourful dreams so take care not to use it with alcohol as nightmares might result.

It is renowned for its ability to produce mildly euphoric states and is therefore considered to be an Aphrodisiac.

Because of its ability to control heat in the body, it can be used by menopausal women and to combat night sweats experienced by people fighting disease.

It is also useful during convalescence. It reduces blood pressure and helps with mood swings and PMS, muscular and joint pain.

TOP TO MIDDLE NOTE WHICH BLENDS WELL WITH: Juniper, Neroli, Marjoram, Lavender, Sandalwood and the Citrus oils.

CAUTIONS: Can be very sedative It is best used in a persons own home so as they will not have to drive after their treatment. It affects concentration and can often have an effect on the practitioner. Generally a safe oil due to its high content of Esters and Alcohols. Not to be used in the first 6 months of pregnancy.

8. CYPRESS – CUPRESSUS SEMPERVIRENS

Extraction from the needles and twigs. Sometimes the cones are used too. The oil is usually pale yellow and has a pleasant, woody, but sweet refreshing odour. Native to Mediterranean Europe it grows wild in many places including France, UK, and the Balkans. There are many varieties of Cypress but *sempervirens* is considered superior and is the oil generally used by Aromatherapists.

PROPERTIES: Antirheumatic, Antiseptic, Antispasmodic, Antsudorific, Astringent, Cicatrisant, Deodorant, Diuretic, Febrifuge, Haemostatic, Hepatic, Insecticide, Sedative, Tonic, and Vasoconstrictor.

USES: Its Vasoconstrictor properties make this an ideal oil to use for any problem relating to the circulatory system where coolness is needed. Particularly good for Haemorrhoids and Varicose veins.

Mix a bath oil or lotion to be applied to the area (not massaged) Mixed with Lavender it is wonderful for healing the perineum after childbirth.

Being a cooling oil it is helpful for hot flushes and pre-menstrual problems.

It may regulate hormone imbalances and has a good effect on ovary dysfunction and painful or heavy periods.

Being antispasmodic it is useful for coughs and asthma. Use a drop on a handkerchief or the pillow at night. It eases the pain of muscular cramps and rheumatism.

It is a tonic to the Circulatory and Digestive system and it helps the liver maintain the regular composition of blood.

Urinary infections respond well with the use of Cypress oil, suitably diluted and massaged into the abdominal area. As it is both Deodorant and Astringent it is helpful for excessive perspiration especially of the feet.

MIDDLE TO BASE NOTE WHICH BLENDS WELL WITH: Lavender, Cedarwood, Pine, Clary Sage, Juniper, Sweet Marjoram and the Citrus oils.

CAUTIONS: Although conclusive evidence is lacking, it may be wise to avoid using this oil in the first 6 months of pregnancy.

9. EUCALYPTUS – EUCALYPTUS GLOBULUS

Steam distilled from the leaves and young twigs of the tree. It produces a pale to dark yellow oil with a strong distinctive antiseptic aroma. The best oils originate in the High Andes.

Cultivated in Southern Europe, North Africa, The Philippines and Australia.

The majority of oils are now produced in Spain, Portugal and Brazil.

PROPERTIES: Analgesic, Anti-catarrhal, Antibacterial, Antifungal, Antirheumatic, Antiseptic, Antiviral, Astringent, Cicatrisant, Decongestant, Expectorant, Febrifuge, Insecticide, Rubifacient, Stimulant, and Vermifuge.

USES: This highly antiseptic oil is so useful for any infections of the respiratory tract such as colds, flu, laryngitis, bronchitis, sore throats, croup, sinusitis, and rhinitis.

Used in a burner it will purify the air to stop infection spreading.

Eucalyptus globulus is also excellent in blends for muscular aches, neuralgia, rheumatism and joint pains.

Its action has a pronounced cooling effect on the body.

Helpful with malaria, measles, diabetes, cystitis, ulcers, sores, burns, blisters, lymph node infections, headaches and neuralgia.

It is used extensively in the pharmaceutical industry, in flavourings and toiletries.

TOP NOTE WHICH, BLENDS WELL WITH: Juniper, Benzoin, Lavender, Bergamot and Melissa.

CAUTIONS: Often rectified. Better not used on highly sensitive people or children, Euc Radiata or Smithii are gentler. Not to be used with homeopathic remedies.

10. EUCALYPTUS – EUCALYPTUS RADIATA
& SMITHII

Both are steam distilled from the leaves and young twigs of the tree and it produces a pale to dark yellow oil with a strong distinctive antiseptic aroma. Their properties are similar to those of Globulus but they are both gentler oils and can be used by the whole family

Smithii is particularly useful as it can be used as a protective measure against infections in the winter months.

The best oils originate in the High Andes. Cultivated in Southern Europe, North Africa, The Philippines and Australia. The majority of oils are now produced in Spain, Portugal and Brazil.

PROPERTIES: Analgesic, Anticatarrhal, Antibacterial, Antifungal, Antirheumatic, Antiseptic, Antiviral, Astringent, Cicatrisant, Decongestant, Expectorant, Febrifuge, Insecticide, Rubifacient, Stimulant, and Vermifuge.

USES: These highly antiseptic oils are useful for any infections of the respiratory tract such as colds, flu, laryngitis, bronchitis, sore throats, croup, sinusitis and rhinitis.

Used in a burner, it will purify the air to stop infection spreading. Both are useful for muscular strain, aches and pains, rheumatism and arthritis.

Each has a pronounced cooling effect on the body.

Helpful with malaria, measles, diabetes, cystitis, ulcers, sores, burns, blisters, lymph node infections, headaches and neuralgia.

Used extensively in the pharmaceutical industry, in flavourings and toiletries.

For children, Euc Radiata or Smithii are recommended. Not to be used with homeopathic remedies.

Radiata is effective when treating upper respiratory tract infections i.e. Mucus conditions, catarrh, sinus and head colds. Direct inhalation is recommended.

TOP NOTE, WHICH BLENDS WELL WITH: Juniper, Benzoin, Lavender, Bergamot and Melissa.

CAUTIONS: None known.

11. SWEET FENNEL – FOENICULUM VULGARE
Var DULCE

Distilled from the crushed seeds, is colourless to pale yellow. It has a strong aroma of anise but is softer with a hint of Camphor.

Sweet Fennel is thought to have originated on the island of Malta. It is now cultivated principally in France, Italy and Greece.

It is closely related to Bitter Fennel (wild), which is not used in Aromatherapy although it has been used medicinally for centuries.

PROPERTIES: Anti-inflammatory, Antiseptic, Antiphlogistic, Antispasmodic, Aperitif, Carminative, Depurative, Diuretic, Emmenagogic, Expectorant, Galactagogic, Laxative, Stimulant, Splenic, Stomachic, Tonic, Vermifuge.

USES: Fennel has long been associated with the digestion and it helps such problems as flatulence, colic, nausea, and indigestion.

It is an ingredient of baby's gripe water. It is considered good for obstruction of the liver, gall bladder, spleen and kidneys.

It is another of the oils that helps poor appetite (Anorexia) It is helpful in detoxifying the body so should help hangovers and can be used for cases of cellulite, obesity and oedema.

It is said that ladies in Ancient Rome ate Fennel to keep themselves slim. It has the reputation of being an appetite depressant.

It promotes lactation and eases mastitis. Fennel contains Estragol and is known to have a beneficial effect on the female reproductive system so it is helpful for regulating the menstrual cycle and easing the symptoms of pre menstrual stress, helps reduce the water retention that so many women experience in the few days before menstruation.

Excellent for cystitis and urinary problems. Considered good for muscular energy.

MIDDLE TO TOP NOTE, WHICH BLENDS WELL WITH: The herbal oils, Lavender, Rose and the Citrus oils.

CAUTIONS: Relatively non-toxic. Not to be used during pregnancy and I have found it better not to use on people who are on the birth control pill or HRT. Nor should it be used on Epileptics.

12. FRANKINCENSE – BOSWELLIA CARTERII
or THURIFERA

Also known as Olibanum it is distilled from the resin from a small tree from China, The Middle East, Ethiopia, Lebanon, and North East Africa.

The gum resin does not occur naturally in the tree but is produced as a protection when the bark is cut and it produces a milky juice, which hardens.

It has a clear refreshing odour, slightly spicy, and the oil is a light golden colour. It improves with age.

PROPERTIES: Analgesic, Antiseptic, Astringent, Carminative, Cicatrisant, Cytophylactic, Digestive, Diuretic, Expectorant, Immuno-stimulant, Sedative, Tonic, Uterine and Vulnerary.

USES: This oil is best known for its ability to deepen and slow the breath and it has a calming effect on the mind and body.

Throughout history, this oil has been used traditionally in the form of incense for religious ceremonies. It produces a state conducive to concentration and meditation.

It is a useful oil to use during a counselling session or at any time when it is necessary to produce a relaxed and trusting atmosphere.

It is considered to be a mind oil as its action on the nervous system produces a feeling of calm. Its comforting action is helpful for anxious or obsessional states linked to the past.

Because of its beneficial effects on breathing, it is useful for treating asthma, laryngitis, bronchitis and coughs. It is invaluable for the treatment of cystitis and urinary infections as well as many digestive problems.

It is found to be effective on wounds, sores, abscesses, ulcers, acne, and inflammation and particularly for its Cicatrisant properties for scarred skin.

Its Astringent properties help balance oily skin conditions. Said to be an effective treatment for nose bleeds.

BASE NOTE, WHICH BLENDS WELL WITH: Geranium. Lavender, Black Pepper, Patchouli and the citrus oils.

CAUTIONS: Although a very safe oil it is not considered suitable for use on children.

13. GERANIUM – PELARGONIUM GRAVEOLENS
or P. ADORATISSIMUM

Steam distilled from the leaves and shoots. The oil is a pale green in colour and has an aroma with the sweetness of Rose and the sharpness of Bergamot.

Originally from South Africa but there are several hundred different species. The best oils come from Renuion. Others come from France, Italy, Corsica, Spain and North Africa.

PROPERTIES: Analgesic, Antiseptic, Antidepressant, Antidiabetic, Astringent, Cicatrisant, Diuretic, Haemostatic, (anti coagulant principle in leaves), Insecticide, Sedative, Tonic, Vulnerary.

USES: Circulatory and Lymphatic, so it is excellent for treating Cellulitis and any sort of congestion in the body.

Helps diabetics and because it is good for circulation it helps with any condition where there is inflammation or infection. It particularly helps with breast problems such as engorgement or mastitis.

It helps kidney functioning so therefore it can help with water retention. It is one of the oils that help hormone regulation so it is useful for problems such as P.M.S. Endometriosis, Infertility and Menopause.

In skin care it is invaluable as it can be used on any skin type and it is especially helpful for Acne and Eczema. As it assists healing, it is good for skin problems and can be used for minor wounds, rashes, burns, ringworm and shingles, Herpes simplex and athlete's foot and it helps alleviate dandruff.

It is often effective in mouth and throat infections, where it acts as an analgesic. Alleviates depression and anxiety and it stimulates the adrenal cortex.

MIDDLE NOTE WHICH BLENDS WELL WITH: Most other essences but especially with the citrus oils.

CAUTIONS: Often falsified with cheaper oils. Very occasionally causes dermatitis in hypersensitive people.

14. GINGER – ZINGIBER OFFICINALE

Extracted from the root by steam distillation, the oil varies from very pale to deep yellow. It has a pungent, warm, spicy aroma and is not really what one expects.

Native to India, China, Java, and Japan, it is also grown in The West Indies, Malaysia and Africa. Most oils are distilled in India, China and the UK.

PROPERTIES: Analgesic, Antiseptic, Anti-spasmodic, Aperitif, Aphrodisiac, Bactericidal, Carminative, Cephalic, Expectorant, Febrifuge, Laxative, Rubifacient, Stimulant, Stomachic, Tonic.

USES: This highly important spice has been used since ancient times and its medicinal and culinary uses are widely recognised throughout the world.

For the digestive system it is renowned for being a stimulant to the whole system. It is excellent for flatulence, colic and nausea and helps with travel and morning sickness.

Ginger is used in traditional Chinese medicine for many purposes but particularly where the body is not efficiently coping with moisture.

A few drops added to a footbath can be very helpful when suffering from colds or flu. For sore throats it is effective as a gargle.

Its Rubifacient qualities make it invaluable for the treatment of arthritis, cramps, stiffness, fibrositis, poor circulation, and water retention.

It has Aphrodisiac properties and it has been used successfully through the ages to help flagging sexual appetites. The Romans used it for eye infections and diseases.

In the Middle Ages it was used to counteract the Black Death. It promotes sweating.

It is used extensively in the food and perfume industries.

BASE NOTE WHICH BLENDS WELL WITH: All the citrus oils, Patchouli, Vetivert and Coriander.

CAUTIONS: Not suitable for highly sensitive skins and it should never be used neat.

15. GRAPEFRUIT – CITRUS PARADISI

Produced by cold expression from the fresh peel. It is greenish / yellow mobile oil with a fresh citrus aroma.

Native to Tropical Asia, it is also grown in California, Florida, Brazil and Israel. Once known as Shaddock fruit it originated in Barbados and Jamaica.

PROPERTIES: Antiseptic, Astringent, Bactericidal, Carminative, Diuretic, Decongestant, Depurative, Stomachic, Stimulant, Tonic.

USES: Like lemon, it is cooling, cleansing, and a decongestant oil A valuable protection against infectious illnesses and can safely be used to combat colds and flu.

Its action on the nervous system makes it a useful anti-depressant, it is recommended for mental and performance stress complaints.

It is another useful oil for muscular fatigue, stiffness and water retention, obesity and cellulitis particularly if blended with one of the Rubifacient oils such as Pine, Vetivert, Black Pepper or Ginger.

It has a stimulant effect on the Lymphatic and Digestive systems so it is a useful cleansing oil, perhaps after too much food or drink.

For congested or oily skin conditions, spots and acne.

This oil is used extensively in desserts, soft drinks and alcoholic beverages.

TOP NOTE WHICH BLENDS WELL WITH: Lavender, Basil, Rose, Benzoin, Geranium and the other citrus oils.

CAUTIONS: Like all the citrus oils it has a short life and oxidizes quickly. Avoid exposure to sun for at least 12 hours after application.

16. JASMINE – JASMINUM OFFICINALE

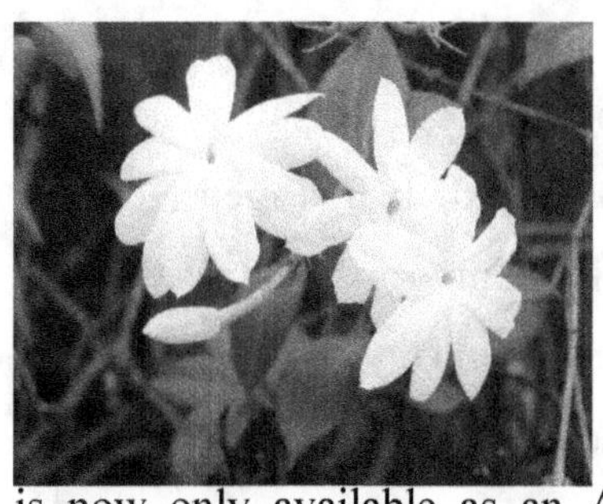

The Essential oil is steam distilled from the Absolute. It is a deep reddish / brown oil with a heady, exotic aroma.

It was once produced by enfleurage and generally speaking it is now only available as an Absolute. It is cultivated in Algeria, Morocco, France, China, Egypt, Italy and Turkey.

PROPERTIES: Anti-depressant, Anti-inflammatory, Antiseptic, Anti-spasmodic, Aphrodisiac, Carminative, Cicatrisant, Expectorant, Galactagogic, Parturient, Sedative, Tonic.

USES: In China the flowers are used to treat hepatitis, liver cirrhosis and dysentery.

Like Rose, this oil is excellent for the reproductive system and is a tonic to the uterus, and will treat menstrual pain.

It is antispasmodic and can effectively be used for relieving spasms either as a result of muscle strain and cramp or of the respiratory system in cases of coughs and breathing difficulties.

It can be used safely on almost any type of skin and has been used in beauty products for centuries.

As an anti-depressant it is most useful in treating cases of apathy, indifference and listlessness.

BASE NOTE WHICH BLENDS WELL WITH: All the other oils.

CAUTIONS: Since the late 1980s essential oil of Jasmine has not been readily available and even the Absolute is extremely expensive. It would probably to be best to use this oil mainly for its fragrance rather than for its therapeutic value as it is unlikely that any oil labelled Essential oil of Jasmine would be so.

17. JUNIPER BERRY – JUNIPERUS COMMUNIS

Distilled from the berry of the Juniper tree, the oil is colourless to pale yellow but it grows darker and thicker with age.

The aroma is similar to Cypress but sharper and more peppery.

Cultivated in Central and Southern Europe, Sweden and Canada.

PROPERTIES: Antiseptic, Antispasmodic, Astringent, Carminative, Cicatrisant, Diuretic, Detoxifying, Emmenogogue, Nervine, Parturient, Rubefacient, Stomachic and Sudorific, Tonic and Vulnerary.

USES: Juniper is excellent for helping complaints of the Genito-urinal system such as cystitis, pyelitis and urinary stones.

It works well to help those who have scanty or missed periods, and also for fluid retention problems before a period.

It is known to protect against infection and it makes a good household disinfectant. It is excellent for exhaustion or over stimulation as it strengthens the nerves.

Helps rid the body of uric acid so is able to ease rheumatic pains, aching joints, gout or sciatica. It is renowned for its detoxifying ability, so it is invaluable for clearing any toxins or mucus out of the body.

For weeping eczema with a carrier oil, preferably Almond, it can be applied every four hours until the symptoms improve.

This oil that has been truly tried and tested as it has been in use since time immemorial. In Tibet, Egypt, Rome and Greece it was used for antiseptic, religious, and culinary purposes

MIDDLE NOTE WHICH BLENDS WELL WITH: Bergamot, Clary Sage, Rosemary, Geranium and the citrus oils.

CAUTIONS: It is important that really pure oil is purchased as the cheaper brands are often adulterated with turpentine. Prolonged use may over stimulate the kidneys.

Not to be used during pregnancy.

18.LAVENDER – LAVENDULA ANGUSTIFOLIA
or LAVENDULA OFFICINALIS

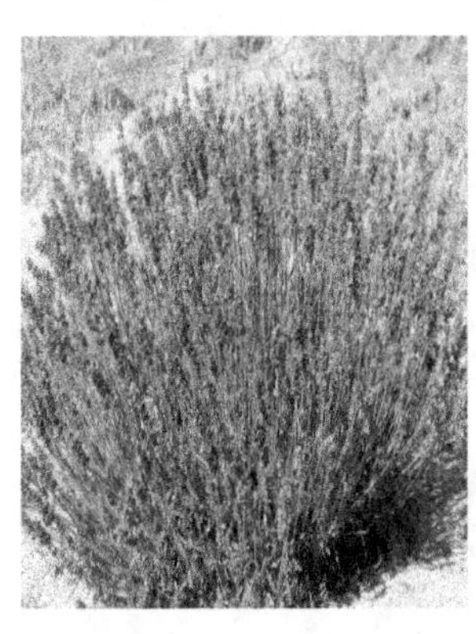

Steam distilled from the flowers, leaves and shoots. The oil is colourless to pale yellow with a sweet, floral-herbaceous aroma.

Indigenous to the Mediterranean, it is now cultivated all over the world. The oil is produced mainly in France also Spain, Italy, England, Australia, Greece and Turkey.

There are many different species of Lavender – stoeches, spike, hidcote, dwarf blues and bowles are just a few.

PROPERTIES: Analgesic, Anticonvulsive, Antidepressant, Anti-inflammatory, Antiseptic, Antispasmodic, Carminative, Chologogic, Cicatrisant, Cordial, Cytophylactic, Diuretic, Emmenagogue, Haemostatic, Hypertensive, Hypotensive, Insecticide, Nervine, Rubifacient, Sedative, Stimulant, Sudorific, Tonic, Vermifuge, Vulnerary.

USES:

Generally regarded as the most versatile essence therapeutically and can be used for almost every conceivable complaint.

It is especially known for its power to help attain deep restful sleep.

Reams have been written about Lavender oil and it is regarded as the most useful oil to have as it can add a pleasant aroma to some of the less pleasant smelling oils.

It is non-toxic and non-irritant. It is one of the few oils that can be used directly onto the skin.

MIDDLE NOTE WHICH BLENDS WELL WITH: All other oils.

CAUTIONS: One of the least toxic oils but care should still be taken as the cheaper Lavendin is often sold as Lavender.

19. LAVENDIN – LAVENDULA FRAGRENS or HYBRIDA

Extraction by steam distillation from the fresh flowering tops of the plant. A hybrid plant developed by crossing *L angustifolia* with Spike lavender *L.latifolia.* Hybridisation occurs naturally as bees convey pollen from one plant to another.

It has a much higher yield than lavender and is easy to cultivate so it is extremely popular with growers and it is often used to adulterate true lavender.

Known in the trade as 'bastard lavender', it does not reproduce. It is cloned to produce more oil per acre and it has a totally different chemical composition to true Lavender. Although it belongs to the same family, it does not have the same therapeutic properties. There are several different cultivars.

It is pale yellow oil and smells very similar to Lavender but because of its Camphor content is sharper and less subtle.

It is primarily cultivated in France, Spain, Italy, Switzerland and Hungary.

It is a relatively, new oil to Aromatherapy and therefore does not have the traditional history of therapeutic uses but the uses can be assessed from the chemical constituents. Cotton and Sea Lavender belong to different botanical families.

PROPERTIES: Analgesic, Antidepressant, Antiseptic, Antiviral, Decongestant, Insecticide, and Tonic.

USES: The properties of Lavendin are similar to Lavender and it is a useful oil to include in your treatments when you don't need the relaxing qualities of Lavender. Good for morning massages.

Good for muscular aches and pains and stiffness both in the bath and in a massage.

It is a refreshing oil and can help with headaches and stuffiness. It is effective to use for colds, sinus problems and catarrh. Because of its Camphor content, it is good for almost any muscular, respiratory or circulatory problems, which are usually helped by Camphor oil. This is a lovely oil to use in burners and diffusers and it is cheaper than Lavender.

MIDDLE TO TOP NOTE WHICH BLENDS WELL WITH: Most other oils.

CAUTIONS: It is best avoided during pregnancy. It is less effective and less therapeutic than Lavender but is often sold as such.

20. LEMON – CITRUS LIMON

Pressed from the rind of lemon, the oil is a pale yellow and has a sharp tangy refreshing smell. The best oils come from India, China, Japan, Spain, Portugal, and California.

PROPERTIES: Antiseptic, Anti-inflammatory, Anti-spasmodic, Astringent, Bactericidal, Carminative, Decongestant, Febrifuge, Hepatic, Hypotensive, Vermifuge and Vulnerary.

USES: Lemon is without doubt one of the most versatile of the oils and used in the right proportions has few contra-indications. Lemon essence neutralises typhus bacillus and staphylococcus in 5 minutes and diptheric bacillus in 20 minutes so it is a powerful bactericide.

It is excellent for external wounds and infections and as a mouthwash for gum infections, gingivitis and mouth ulcers. For the removal of corns, warts and verrucas (2 drops Lemon oil, 10 drops cider vinegar).

It helps with digestive problems. Cleanses the blood and acts as a lymphatic decongestant so useful on cellulite, for obesity, high blood pressure, cholesterol, and arteriosclerosis.

It is worth noting that Lemon juice counteracts acidity in the body, citric acid neutralizes during digestion giving rise to carbonates and bicarbonates of potassium and calcium, which helps maintain alkalinity in the system.

Other uses include treatment for dandruff, P.M.T. migraine, insect and snake bites.

Excellent for greasy skin problems. Cellulite and circulatory conditions like chilblains respond well to this oil. Eases bronchial and sinus infections. Use for sprains, muscular aches and pains and rheumatism.

TOP NOTE, WHICH BLENDS WELL WITH: Lavender, Ylang Ylang, Frankincense, Chamomile and Ginger. Other citrus oils.

CAUTIONS: Lemon oil does not keep well and careful storage is necessary. If it is not fresh it can irritate the skin. It should only be used in small proportions and is best mixed with another oil. It is Phototoxic so the skin should not be exposed to sunlight after use.

21. LEMONGRASS – CYMBOPOGON CITRATUS

Steam distilled from the fresh and partially dried grass, the oil in yellow / brown and has a strong lemon aroma.

There are several varieties of lemongrass but cymbopogon citratus is recommended for massage treatments.

It is native to tropical Asia and is cultivated in India, Sri Lanka, Indonesia, Africa, Madagascar, The Seychelles, South and tropical North America.

PROPERTIES: Analgesic, Antidepressant, Antiseptic, Astringent, Bactericidal, Carminative, Deodorant, Febrifuge, Fungicidal, Galactagogic, Insecticide, Nervine, Sedative, and Tonic.

USES: As it acts as a sedative on the central nervous system, it is useful for exhaustion and stress-related conditions.

Can be used to relieve jet lag, clears headaches, and fatigue.

It is calming too for the digestive system and particularly useful for gastro-enteritis and colitis.

Used in traditional Indian medicine as a febrifuge.

It can be used for infectious illness and fevers.

It is helpful for strengthening muscle tone, slack tissue, and poor circulation as it tones the muscles.

In very small proportions it is useful for congested and greasy skin conditions, acne, excessive perspiration and athlete's foot.

Used extensively to flavour Eastern cooking. It is a mild insect repellent.

TOP NOTE, WHICH BLENDS WELL WITH: Lavender, Basil, Rosemary, Jasmine, Palmarosa, Neroli, Tea Tree and Ylang Ylang.

CAUTIONS: Use only in low dosage as it can be an irritant on sensitive skins. Do not use during pregnancy.

22. MANDARIN – CITRUS MADURENSIS
or C RETICULATA

Expressed from the peel of the fruit, it has a sweet, tangy aroma. It is a golden yellow oil with a blue / violet luminosity. Produced in South America mainly Brazil, China, Italy, California and the Mediterranean.

PROPERTIES: Antiseptic, Anti-fungal, Anti-spasmodic, Carminative, Chologogic, Cytophylactic, Depurative, Digestive, Diuretic, Sedative, Tonic.

USES: A good tonic for the digestive system, it stimulates appetite and helps to regulate the metabolic processes. Aids in the secretion of bile as it has a stimulating effect on the liver.

It can be safely used on young children. It is useful for over-active or hyperactive youngsters or anyone who needs balancing and calming. Try a couple of drops in their evening bath.

Nice too for the elderly, it has an uplifting quality and is therefore good for low spirits and convalescence.

Sedative to the nervous system and helps banish depression, therefore excellent for treating PMS particularly if mixed with Clary sage or Chamomile.

Mandarin is a gentle oil and can be used safely during pregnancy.

Mixed with Lavender, Neroli or Chamomile in a good base oil will prevent stretch marks during pregnancy.

TOP TO MIDDLE NOTE WHICH BLENDS WELL WITH: Lavender, Chamomile, Black pepper, Petigrain, Marjoram, Palmarosa, Rose, and the other Citrus oils.

CAUTIONS: May be phototoxic, so is best not used if going into strong sunlight. It is often adulterated and it deteriorates quickly.

23. SWEET MARJORAM – ORIGANUM MAJORANA
or MAJORANA HORTENSIS

Produced by steam distillation of the dried flowering Herb, the oil is a pale yellow, mobile liquid, which darkens with age. It has a warm, woody aroma with a hint of Camphor.

There are several varieties of Marjoram. Other varieties include O. onites (Pot marjoram), Thymus mastichino (Wild marjoram) and O. vulgare (Origanum), which is also a wild plant from which Origanum Essential oil, is extracted.

Sweet Marjoram is produced in France, Tunisia, Morocco, Egypt, Bulgaria, Hungary and Germany.

PROPERTIES: Analgesic, Anaphrodisiac, Antiseptic, Antispasmodic, Antiviral, Bactericidal, Carminative, Cephalic, Cordial, Digestive, Diuretic, Emmenagogic, Expectorant, Hypotensive, Laxative, Nervine, Sedative, Stomachic, Tonic, Vasodilator, Vulnerary.

USES: Well known as a culinary Herb for flavouring, it has been used for centuries. It was used for medicinal purposes in Ancient Greece.

It is extremely helpful with chest infections, colds, asthma, sinusitis and earaches.

It is a relaxing oil and mixed with Lavender or Sweet Orange will help insomnia.

For all stress-related conditions, hypertension, headaches, migraine and nervous tension. Used to help prevent bedwetting and excellent for hyperactivity in children.

It helps regulate the menstrual cycle and relieves painful periods. However it has the reputation for quelling sexual desire. It is said to help regulate the thyroid.

It is a good circulatory oil, it is warming so therefore it will help with stiffness, rheumatism, arthritis, aches and pains, strains and bruising.

Mixed with Rosemary or Sage, it helps prevent falling hair and will keep the scalp healthy.

MIDDLE NOTE, WHICH BLENDS WELL WITH: Lavender, Orange, Bergamot, Cedarwood, Rosemary, Cypress and Ylang Ylang.

CAUTIONS: It is best not to use this oil during the first 6 months of pregnancy mainly because of the variety of qualities available. Over use could cause drowsiness.

24. MAY CHANG – LITSEA CUBEBA

The essential oil is steam distilled from the fruits of a small tropical tree and the fruit is described as looking similar to peppers.

It is chemically very like Lemongrass and Melissa, and the therapeutic effects are similar to Lemongrass.

The oil is pale yellow and it has a more truly lemon smell than either Melissa or Lemongrass but with a fruity tang.

It belongs to the same family as the laurel, rosewood and cinnamon tree. Native to Asia especially China, it is cultivated in Taiwan and Japan.

PROPERTIES: Anti-depressant, Anti-inflammatory, Antiseptic, Astringent, Carminative, Cordial, Deodorant, Digestive, Galactagogic, Hypotensive, Insecticide, Stimulant, Stomachic, Tonic.

USES: Studies in China have confirmed its anti-arrhythmic properties. It is suggested that it may have a beneficial effect on coronary heart disease.

Also recognised for treating dysmenorrhoea, stomach cramps, lower back pain and headaches.

It is an effective bronchodilator and can be used for problems of the respiratory system such as coughs, bronchitis and asthma.

As an anti-depressant, calming and balancing and it is most useful in treating cases of apathy, listlessness and indifference as it is a truly uplifting smell. It is said to help reduce anger.

It has a tonic and astringent effect on the skin making it useful for the treatment of oily skin and acne problems.

TOP NOTE WHICH BLENDS WELL WITH: Almost all other oils.

CAUTIONS: Non-toxic and generally non-irritant.

25. MELISSA – MELISSA OFFICINALIS

Commonly known as balm or lemon balm this oil is steam distilled from the leaves and tops of the plant. It is a pale lemon oil with a distinct warm, lemon aroma.

It is a common plant and grows wild in many places in Europe but the yield of essential oil is very small so Melissa True is a very costly oil.

It is native to the Mediterranean and is now common throughout Europe, Asia, USA, N Africa and Russia. The oil is produced almost exclusively in France. The Romans introduced it into England nearly two thousand years ago.

PROPERTIES: Anti-depressant, Antiseptic, Antispasmodic, Bactericidal, Carminative, Cordial, Emmenagogic, Febrifuge, Hypertensive, Nervine, Sedative, Stomachic, Sudorific, Tonic, Uterine, Vermifuge.

USES: Soothing to mind and body this oil is particularly associated with nervous disorders, the heart and the emotions so it acts as a tonic to the nervous system.

It helps in cases of people suffering from melancholy, bereavement or shock. This is one of the best oils for treating high blood pressure.

Will help palpitations and dizziness.

It is calming to the digestive system and aids indigestion and flatulence.

It helps regulate the menstrual cycle so this is an oil well employed in cases of infertility caused by scanty or irregular periods.

It is effective mixed with Chamomile in some cases of allergies and sensitivities but a healing crisis may sometimes occur. Used as a remedy for wasp and bee stings.

It is used extensively as a fragrance component in toiletries, cosmetics, food and drink flavouring and perfumes.

MIDDLE NOTE WHICH BLENDS WELL WITH: Rose, Geranium, Lavender and the citrus oils.

CAUTIONS: Often falsified with Lemongrass, lemon or citronella. Can be a skin irritant to those with delicate skin so always use in very low concentrates. Always use carefully.

26. NEROLI – CITRUS AURANTIUM AMARA

Distilled from the blossom of the bitter orange tree. The oil is a dark yellow viscous liquid with a fresh, sweet, floral aroma.

Native to the Far East, but grown in North Africa, the Mediterranean and the USA. Producers of the oil include Tunisia, France and Sicily.

An Absolute is also produced by solvent extraction.

PROPERTIES: Antidepressant, Antiseptic, Antispasmodic, Aphrodisiac, Bactericidal, Carminative, Cicatrisant, Cordial, Digestive, Fungicide, Stimulant, Tonic.

USES: Probably the best oil for depression, shock and anxiety. It can be used for grief, nervous tension and is particularly valuable during pregnancy and labour.

For insomnia, this is a gentle oil that induces peaceful sleep.

It is excellent for poor circulation and is a natural blood cleanser.

Helps with menopausal problems and PMS. Its antispasmodic properties make it useful for painful periods and ovulation pain.

It is calming to the digestive system, diarrhoea, flatulence, spasms, etc.

Good for mature and sensitive skins, thread veins and stretch marks particularly if mixed with Frankincense.

BASE NOTE WHICH BLENDS WELL WITH: Chamomile, Benzoin, Clary Sage and all the Citrus oils.

CAUTIONS: A safe non-toxic oil, but because of the high price is often adulterated with Petigrain.

It is phototoxic and should be stored carefully as it deteriorates when exposed to light and air.

27. NIAOULI – MELALEUCA VIRIDIFLORA

One of the many Melaleucas, this oil is distilled from the fresh leaves and twigs of the tree. It is a very liquid colourless to pale yellow and is similar to Cajuput (M leucadendron).

It has a clean, rather sweet, antiseptic aroma, balsamic with a hint of Camphor.

It is native to Australia, New Caledonia and The French Pacific Islands. The oil is produced in Australia and Tasmania.
Usually rectified to remove irritant aldehydes.

PROPERTIES: Analgesic, Anti-catarrhal, Antiseptic, Bactericidal, Cicatrisant, Decongestant, Expectorant, Stimulant, Vermifuge, Vulnerary.

USES: An immune supporting oil, it is highly antiseptic so it is useful for infections, colds, dental abscesses, flu and fever. It can be used as a gargle.

Infection of the Genito-Urinary system respond well to this oil. Add a few drops to a bidet or sitz bath for cystitis, urinary infection, leucorrhoea or puritis.

Helps with joint and muscle pain, rheumatism and poor circulation.

Indicated for any problem of the respiratory system, asthma, bronchitis, catarrh, coughs, sinusitis, sore throat, and whooping cough.

Clears the head and said to aid concentration.

In skin care, it is useful for oily conditions and acne but also for wounds, cuts, ulcers and bites. It helps relieve itching.

TOP NOTE, WHICH BLENDS WELL WITH: Lavender, Neroli, Sandalwood and Geranium.

CAUTIONS: None known but the oil is sometimes adulterated. Avoid in the first 6 months of pregnancy.

28. ORANGE – CITRUS VULGARIS / AURANTIUM / CINESIS

Usually expressed, but sometimes steam distilled from the peel of the orange. The oil has a sweet, gentle fruity aroma and it should be a pale orange colour that goes brown as it deteriorates.

Native to China, it is now grown extensively in America, The Mediterranean and Israel. There are many varieties of orange trees and new ones often appear.

Bitter Orange (var. Amara) is a lovely oil but should be reserved for use in a burner or for pot pourri.

PROPERTIES: Antidepressant, Anti-inflammatory, Antiseptic, Bactericidal, Carminative, Digestive, Fungicidal, Hypotensive, Sedative, Stimulant, Stomachic, Tonic.

USES: Orange is a cheerful oil, it can lift depression and boredom and encourage a positive outlook. It is useful for lethargic teenagers or children. Good for circulatory problems and general aches and pains.

It is extremely useful for regulating the digestive system and I have found it helps IBS. In fact it will calm a nervous stomach and encourages the production of bile. It is also said to be a detoxifying oil. It is said to aid the absorption of vitamin C and could therefore be used to help fight off viral infections .

A lovely oil mixed with hazelnut, almond and wheatgerm base for rejuvenating skin and combating wrinkles. Especially good after an overdose of sun. It is useful for eczema and dermatitis.

TOP NOTE WHICH BLENDS WELL WITH: The Herbal and Citrus oils, Cypress, Clary sage, Frankincense, Juniper, Lavender, Petigrain, Geranium and Rose.

CAUTIONS: Difficult to preserve well. It should be kept in the dark and cool. The Oranges provided for Essential oil must be organically grown and be as natural and untampered with as possible

29. PALMAROSA – CYMBOPOGON MARTINII

Steam distilled from the wild grass after it has been dried. It is pale yellow oil and has a sweet floral odour, a mixture of Rose and Geranium.

It comes from the same family as Citronella and Lemongrass and was once known as Indian Geranium. It is native India and Pakistan, now grown in Africa, Indonesia, Java, Brazil and the Comoro islands.

It is one of the oils used to adulterate other oils, especially Rose and Geranium for obvious reasons.

PROPERTIES: Antiseptic, Antiviral, Bactericide, Cytophylactic, Digestive, Febrifuge, and Tonic.

USES: A valuable skin care oil, used with almond oil it is hydrating and stimulating.

It is known to have cell regenerative properties and it regulates sebum production.

This makes it useful for almost any skin condition.

It is a nerve relaxant and is useful for nervous exhaustion and stress-related conditions.

As a digestive stimulant it can have a beneficial effect on poor appetite and may be helpful for people suffering from Anorexia nervosa.

Has been used successfully when the body is overheated and feverish.

This is an oil, which is used extensively in the perfume industry, and it is the ingredient of many soaps and cosmetics and is also used as a flavouring for tobacco.

TOP NOTE WHICH BLENDS WELL WITH: Geranium, Sandalwood, Cedarwood, all of the Citrus and Floral oils.

CAUTIONS: There seems to be no known contra-indications to this oil. Perhaps it would be wise not to use it on anyone known to have an allergy / sensitivity to cosmetics and perfumes.

30. PATCHOULI – POGOSTEMON CABLIN

Distilled from the leaves and shoots after they have been sun dried.

The oil can vary from liquid and transparent to thick yellow / brown with a green tinge. It has an earthy, musty and pungent aroma.

The oils are mainly produced in Sumatra, India, China, Japan, and the USA.

PROPERTIES: Antidepressant, Antiseptic, Antiviral, Anti-inflammatory, Aphrodisiac, Astringent, Diuretic, Cicatrisant, Nervine, Sedative, Tonic, Vulnerary.

USES: Patchouli has been used as a perfume for centuries. It is a natural fixative.

It is one of the oils that have a reputation as an Aphrodisiac perhaps because of its action on the Endocrine glands.

It is sedative in high doses and stimulating in small ones, so although it is a Base note it is perhaps better not used at night as the effect of stimulation or sedation, not only depends on the dose but also on the state of the individual.

It is recommended for many skin conditions such as herpes simplex, bedsores, impetigo, acne, burns, seborrhoea, eczema, and haemorrhoids. It is a skin rejuvenator, so is excellent for elderly skin.

It has an antidepressant effect and has been used in treatments of obesity, possibly because of reports (unsubstantiated) that it induces loss of appetite and because it reduces water retention

It has a balancing effect on the digestive system so can be used for both diarrhoea and constipation.

BASE NOTE WHICH BLENDS WELL WITH: Bergamot, Clove, Lavender, Rose, Clary Sage, Cedarwood, Black pepper and Lemongrass.

CAUTIONS: This oil is often adulterated so get to know it well.

31. PEPPERMINT – MENTHA PIPERITA

Steam distilled from the flowering Herb, the oil is a pale green / yellow with a highly penetrating mint odour. It was known in the 17th century England.

It is cultivated worldwide. Produced mainly in France, Bulgaria, Russia, USA, Italy, Hungary, Morocco, China and the UK.

There are a number of mint species including M Arvensis and M Spicata. Only the latter is sometimes used in Aromatherapy.

PROPERTIES: Anaesthetic,   Analgesic,   Antigalactigogic, Antiseptic, Antispasmodic, Astringent, Antiviral, Carminative, Cephalic,   Chologogic,   Cordial,   Decongestant,   Digestive, Emmenagogic, Expectorant, Febrifuge, Hepatic, Nervine, Stimulant, Stomachic, Sudorific, Vasoconstrictor, Vermifuge.

USES: Excellent oil for mental fatigue, anger, hysteria and nervous tension.

It is useful for relaxing the stomach so can be used for acute problems of diarrhoea and constipation, nausea, flatulence, gallstones and food poisoning.

Its cooling and pain relieving actions make it useful for migraine headaches, toothache, aching limbs, joints and neuralgia. Useful in fever cases and being a decongestant for colds and flu with sinus or mucus problems.

For asthma problems because it is antispasmodic, locally applied (diluted) or in a burner, not inhaled directly.

With skin problems such as acne, dermatitis, ringworm and scabies, used in small proportion will help the irritation and infection.

Lovely for aching feet.

TOP NOTE, WHICH BLENDS WELL WITH: Lavender, Neroli, Benzoin, Mandarin, Rosemary and Niaouli.

CAUTIONS: Peppermint is a powerful oil and dosage should always be small as it can cause skin sensitivity.

Best used in infusers and applied locally rather than for massage.

Best avoided by nursing mothers since it could discourage the flow of milk.

32. PETIGRAIN – CITRUS AURANTIUM

Distilled from the leaves, twigs and sometimes the unripe fruit of the Orange tree, it has a clean, green aroma with a hint of orange.

It is a native to Central Asia but the oil is now grown and produced in Mediterranean countries such as Italy, Spain, Egypt, Tunisia and France. The best oil comes from Grasse in France but little is produced there now.

An inferior oil is also produced in Paraguay.

PROPERTIES: Antidepressant, Antiseptic, Antispasmodic, Digestive, Nervine, Sedative, Stimulant, Stomachic, Tonic

USES: The properties of Petigrain are very similar to Neroli and can be used effectively for anxiety, insomnia, strain and tension.

It slows the body down, eases breathing and relaxes muscle spasms.

Use in cases of extreme fatigue. It is helpful for backache and after long journeys.

Helpful after illness as it acts as a mild immuno-stimulant. It encourages resistance to illness.

It helps reduce skin blemishes, greasy skin conditions and acne and is nice to use in a facial sauna.

It is good for oedema and general puffiness brought on by PMS or digestive disorders such as flatulence or dyspepsia.

MIDDLE TO TOP NOTE WHICH BLENDS WELL WITH: The other citrus oils, Geranium, Rosemary, Sandalwood, Ylang Ylang, Lavender, Cedarwood.

CAUTIONS: As with other citrus oils it has a short life and should be stored carefully. Can be safely used for children in small doses.

Often Petigrain is sold as the more expensive Neroli.

33. PINE – PINUS SYLVESTRIS

There are many different species of Pine but we only use *Sylvestris* in Aromatherapy.

The oil is extracted from the pine needles (leaves) and sometimes the twigs and cones. It is distilled and the oil varies from almost colourless to yellow.

It has a fresh, strong, clean aroma with a balsamic tone.

It comes mainly from Russia, Siberia, North America and Western and Northern Europe. It was once common in Scotland but during the time of wooden sailing ships it was used extensively resulting in the depletion of the forests.

PROPERTIES: Antiphlogistic, Antiseptic, Decongestant, Diuretic, Expectorant, Rubifacient, Sudorific, Stimulant, Tonic.

USES: In ancient civilisations its curative properties were recognised particularly for pulmonary complaints like bronchitis, tuberculosis and pneumonia. Inhalation was primarily used.

At the first sign of viral infection use Pine, Eucalyptus and Niaouli (diluted of course) to massage the chest and back. It is highly antiseptic so can be used to treat infection of almost any kind.

It is recommended for muscle and joint pains and it is useful to use in compresses for sciatica, lumbago, gout and arthritis.

It is a refreshing and stimulating oil so is useful as an uplifting fragrance especially if used in a burner. Some people find it relaxing.

Can be used for PMS, digestive problems, male sexual disorders and as an insecticide.

It is a gentle kidney cleanser and known to be effective with cystitis.

It has a heating effect so it can help poor peripheral circulation.

MIDDLE NOTE, WHICH BLENDS WELL WITH: Lavender, Cedarwood, Clove, Niaouli, and Eucalyptus.

CAUTIONS: May irritate sensitive skins. Not advisable in early pregnancy.

34. RAVENSARA – RAVENSARA AROMATICA

Extracted and steam distilled from the young leafy twigs of a tall, leafy evergreen tree.

The plant has similarities to the Laurel (Laurus nobilis).

It has a red / grey bark and is commonly known as Madagascar Spice or nutmeg, Allspice or Clove nut (Philippe Mailhebiau ' Poirtrait in oils').

All parts of the tree are strongly aromatic. It has a soft spicy, antiseptic smell and is almost colourless. It is native to Madagascar but it is also cultivated in Reunion and Mauritius.

PROPERTIES: Antibacterial, Antivirol, Antifungal, Anti-inflammatory, Carminative, Detoxicant, Expectorant, Stomachic, Tonic (nerve).

USES: Reputed by ancient tribes to be a panacea against bodily and mental ills, it is useful for almost any complaint.

In Madagascar all parts of the part have been used in traditional medicine. Useful for flu as it has highly anti-infectious properties and is an immuno-stimulant.

It should be used at the first sign of chills, shivers or overtiredness. All respiratory tract infections respond well to it. Use especially for bronchitis, rhinitis, sinusitis, whooping cough and TB.

A combination of Cham Roman, Peppermint, Eucalyptus radiata and Lavender will treat shingles and herpes effectively.

It is a mental and physical stimulant and is wonderful for treating fatigue of any sort. It relieves depression and anxiety and is good for people with low self-esteem and those lacking in confidence, those who don't enjoy life and lack motivation or aim in their lives.

It seems to help those who feel ready for a change in life, but it can be disturbing for those who are perhaps not so ready. It is particularly good applied to the spinal area for stress or tension pain in that area.

A muscle relaxant, it will help joint and muscle pain and mixed with Thymus vulgaris c. v. linalool, is particularly good for rheumatoid arthritis.

MIDDLE NOTE WHICH BLENDS WELL WITH: All other oils.

CAUTIONS: It can be used safely on sensitive people and all skin types.

35. ROSE – ROSA DAMASCENA

Probably the first flower from which essential oil was distilled in 10th

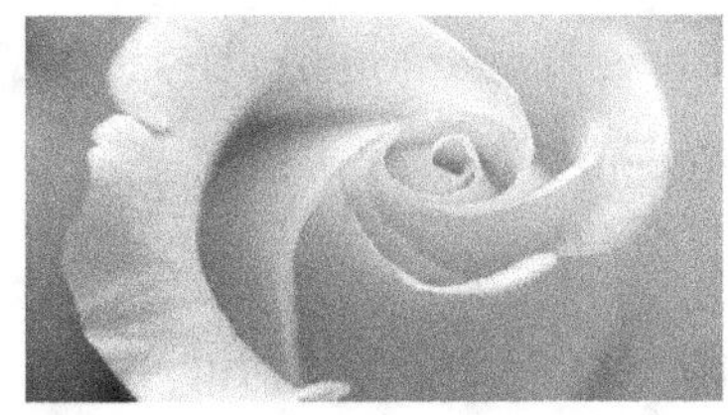

century Persia. Rose Damascena is distilled or enfleuraged from the petals and stamens. It takes 30 roses to produce 1 drop of Bulgarian Rose Otto extracted from the Damascena rose.

The oil varies in colour and is a very pale green / yellow. The very best Rose Otto comes from Bulgaria but fine oil is also produced in Turkey, Morocco, and China. India produces mainly rose water and *Aytar, which is a mixture of Rose and Sandalwood essential oil.* It is not necessary to describe its fragrance, it is probably the best known in the world.

Another Rose that is used is *Centifolia* which is mainly cultivated in Grasse in S France and N Africa and it is solvent extracted to produce an Absolute.

PROPERTIES: Antidepressent, Antiseptic, Antispasmodic, Antiviral, Aphrodisiac, Astringent, Bactericidal, Cicatrisant, Depurative, Emmenagogue, Haemostatic, Hepatic, Laxative, Sedative, Stomachic, Tonic.

USES: Rose oil has so many uses but without doubt it is most powerful when dealing with menstrual and gynaecological problems.

It is invaluable for PMS, postnatal depression, cleansing, regulating, and toning the uterus.

Because of its action on the nervous, vascular and digestive systems it is wonderful for any stress-related conditions such as depression, grief, nervous tension, peptic ulcers, heart disease, IBS, frigidity and male impotence.

It is a good oil for improving circulation and can be helpful for cellulite.

Rose is used for sore or puffy eyes, a compress for skin ulcers and a gargle for a sore throat. It was a constituent of one of the earliest cold creams and it was recorded in a recipe by Galen in the 2nd century.

It is excellent for mature skin, wrinkles and broken capillaries. Because its action is said to increase the production of bile it may be useful in cases of jaundice. Many liqueurs, yoghurts, jams and fruit drinks are flavoured with Rose essential oil.

BASE NOTE WHICH BLENDS WELL WITH: Almost every oil and particularly well with the citrus and herbal oils. There are no known Contra-indications.

CAUTIONS: None known.

36. ROSEMARY – ROSEMARINUS OFFICINALIS

Distilled from the flowering tops, stems, and leaves of the plant. The oil is colourless to pale yellow / green.

It should smell Camphory with a hint of incense and honey.

The best oils come from North Africa, mainly Tunisia, but other good oils are produced in Mediterranean countries and Yugoslavia.

PROPERTIES: Analgesic, Antidepressant, Antiseptic, Antispasmodic, Astringent, Carminative, Cephalic, Chologogic, Cicatrisant, Decongestant, Diuretic, Emmenogogue, Hepatic, Hypertensive, Nervine, Stimulant, Stomatic, Sudorfic, Tonic, and Vulnerary.

USES: In Ancient Greece Rosemary was a symbol of love and death. It has been used for centuries in hair and beauty products.

It has a tonic effect on dark hair and it helps it to retain its colour.

It is useful for treating fatigue and headaches as it has the ability to enliven the brain cells.

Mixed with Basil, it assists mental clarity and alertness.

It has analgesic properties so it aids problems such as arthritis, joint pain, sprains, colds and flu and over tired muscles.

It is a valuable heart tonic and cardiac stimulant, normalising low blood pressure.

It is excellent for digestive problems and is particularly good for constipation, as it seems to stimulate peristalsis.

Helps relieve congestion generally in the body so helps with cellulite, fluid retention and obesity.

MIDDLE NOTE, WHICH BLENDS WELL WITH: Geranium, Melissa, Peppermint, Lavender, Basil and Ginger.

CAUTIONS: There are many different varieties of Rosemary oil, and it's best to stick to the officinalis as the borneol, cineole and verbone are a different chemical makeup.

Because Rosemary is highly stimulating it may not be suitable for people with high blood pressure and should be avoided by epileptics.

It is best avoided during pregnancy.

37. SANDALWOOD – SANTALUM ALBUM

Obtained by distillation from the heartwood and roots of the tree, as it matures it changes from a pale yellow to a deep green or amber colour.

It has a soft, woody balsamic odour.

The very best oils come from Mysore and India is responsible for most of the world's production.

It is also produced in Sri Lanka, Indonesia, Taiwan and some oil is distilled in the USA and Europe. About 90% of oil produced is used in the perfume industry.

PROPERTIES: Antidepressant, Antiphlogistic, Antiseptic, Antispasmodic, Aphrodisiac, Astringent, Bactericidal, Carminative, Cicatrisant, Diuretic, Expectorant, Fungicidal, Insecticidal, Sedative, Tonic.

USES: Used for centuries this oil is excellent for the respiratory system and helps with the treatment of chest infections, sore throats and dry coughs.

Effective for catarrhal problems and for the relief of kidney complaints and cystitis. It is very relaxing and because of its aphrodisiac qualities can relieve problems such as frigidity and impotence.

It was used in the past for infections of the genitals and sexually transmitted diseases. Eases cystitis.

It is good for inflammation or the skin, allergic reaction, abscesses, eczema and acne. It has its best results on dry skin conditions.

Used at night, it is helpful for insomnia and can ease nervous tension and stress-related problems. It is good to use in a burner for meditation and relaxation.

As a hormone regulator, it is useful for problems related to menstruation. It has a traditional use in Chinese medicine for the heart, gall bladder and kidneys. It is used extensively in perfumes and is an excellent fixative.

BASE NOTE, WHICH BLENDS WELL WITH: Benzoin, Basil, Bergamot, Black Pepper, Geranium, Lavender, Patchouli, Neroli, Myrrh, Ylang Ylang Vetivert.

CAUTIONS: A safe non-toxic oil but it is often adulterated. If you are concerned with environmental issues it is best to avoid using this oil. Production has caused wide-scale destruction of many forests. Other oils that have similar therapeutic properties.

38. TEA TREE – MELALEUCA ALTERNIFOLIA

Distilled from the leaves of the tree, the oil is a very pale yellow green. It has a spicy, antiseptic aroma. It is only grown in New South Wales Australia.

PROPERTIES: Antifungal,   Anti-inflammatory,   Antiseptic, Antiviral, Cicatrisant, Cytophylatic, Decongestant, and Vulnerary.

USES: Because this oil is 11-12 times more antiseptic than carbolic acid or phenol, it is effective against a range of bacterial, viral and fungal conditions.

It is used widely in disinfectant, toothpaste, and gargles. It has the added advantage of being both hypoallergenic and non-toxic.

It is useful in treating colds and flu and alleviates sore throats, tonsillitis, and gum disease. It eases bronchitis and congestion.

It calms diarrhoea and relieves gastro-enteritis, it is useful in treating Candida albicans. It is invaluable for treating complaints of the Genito-urinary system such as thrush, trichomonal, cystitis and vaginitis. Is effective for skin problems, particularly boils, acne, infected wounds and burns or fungal problems such as athlete's foot.

It is also an extremely effective insect repellent.

Although Tea Tree is relatively new oil in terms of Aromatherapy, the natives of Australia have used it for centuries. This oil has been extensively researched and documented.

In 1980 it was subjected to stringent testing and it was found that a solution 4 parts Essential oil to 1000 parts water, used against virulent organisms such as Staphylococus aureas and Candida Albicans showed that after testing on the 7th, 21st and 35th days there was no growth detected in the organism. This suggests that when the body is threatened, Tea Tree has the ability to support the Immune response.

TOP TO MIDDLE NOTE, WHICH BLENDS WELL WITH: Lavender, Geranium, Rosemary, and the spice oils particularly Clove.

CAUTIONS: Slight possibility of irritation on sensitive skin.

39. VETIVERT – VETIVERIA ZIZANOIDES

Steam distilled from the scented grass roots after drying, the oil is a deep amber viscous liquid with a heavy, spicy yet earthy aroma.

Native to India, Indonesia and Sri Lanka, the oil is mainly produced in Java, Haiti, Europe and the USA. The best oil comes from Reunion. It is related to Lemongrass, Palmarosa and Citronella.

PROPERTIES: Antiseptic, Antispasmodic, Cytophylactic, Depurative, Rubifacient, Sedative, Stimulant, Tonic, Vermifuge, Vulnerary.

USES: An invaluable oil for the nervous system – depression, tension, insomnia, hysteria, irritability, anger, apprehension and worry. A good grounding oil and for those needing physical energy. Cooling and strengthening.

Used for PMS and menopausal symptoms because of its regulatory action on the hormonal secretion oestrogen and progesterone. It stimulates pancreatic secretion, which may indicate it for the use on people suffering from Diabetes.

Strengthens connective tissue, chronic joint hypermobility, wrinkles and stretch marks.

Said to be an Aphrodisiac, it is traditionally linked to the goddess Aphrodite. Because so many sexual disorders are linked to an anxious mind and panicking under stress (premature ejaculation and frigidity) it can help focus on the physical, sensuous aspect of lovemaking.

Its best and most useful effects are as an insect repellent.

In Russia, small sachets of essential oil of Vetivert were sewn into the linings of expensive fur coats as it is effective against moths. A few drops on a piece of blotting paper or cotton wool can be kept amongst clothing. Used as a fixative in perfumes.

BASE NOTE, WHICH BLENDS WELL WITH: Rose, Patchouli, Geranium, Grapefruit, Lemon, Lavender, Ylang Ylang.

CAUTIONS: None known.

40. YLANG YLANG – CANANGA ODORATA

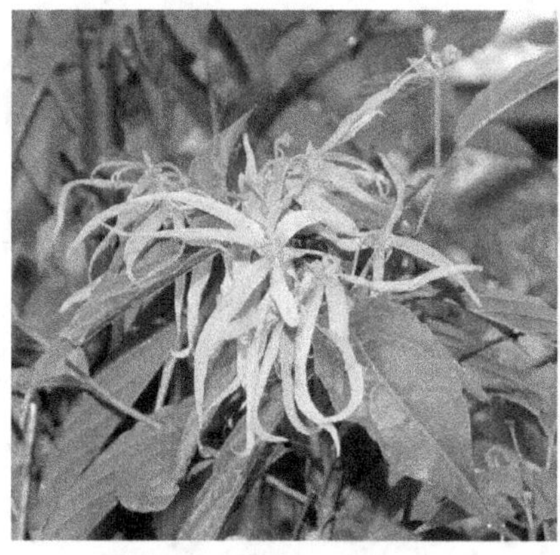

Distilled from the flowers (the name means flower of flowers in Malay) the oil is colourless to pale yellow.

It has a heavy sweet aroma.

The best oils come from Madagascar, Reunion and the Comoro Islands, others come from the Philippines, Java and Sumatra.

PROPERTIES: Antiseptic, Antidepressant, Aphrodisiac, Hypotensive, Sedative.

USES: This oil is best known for its ability to reduce heart rate (tachicardia) and rapid breathing (hyperpnoea). It is excellent to use in cases of shock, anger, fear, overwork, frustration (including sexual) or anxiety and it helps reduce high blood pressure.

Its antidepressant and Aphrodisiac qualities are well known in helping with sexual problems such as impotence and frigidity.

It is an oil that is widely used in the perfume and cosmetic industry and is known to be a scalp tonic. In the Victorian age, the oil was used in a popular hair treatment, Macassar oil, due to its stimulating effect on the scalp, encouraging hair growth.

Mixed with Coconut oil it was used by the natives of the Philippine islands to protect their hair and their skin when they swam. They called it Borri-borri and also used it to avoid the bites of snakes and insects.

BASE NOTE WHICH BLENDS WELL WITH: It blends beautifully with Lemon and Bergamot, both of which help reduce the slightly sweet sickly aroma that can sometimes induce nausea and headaches. Rosemary, Jasmine, Lavender and Sandalwood.

CAUTIONS: Can cause headaches and nausea. Should not be used on inflamed skin conditions.

THE CARRIER OILS

The Carrier oils are the oily base oils into which we mix our essential oils. They are fixed oils. A fixed oil is a compound of glycerol and fatty acid – a Glyceride is called fixed, to distinguish it from the essential oils which evaporate when warmed.

Because they easily deteriorate on exposure to air they should be kept cool and always have the tops replaced immediately after use.

Each practitioner has their own preferences of base oil. Grapeseed and Coconut are my favourites, both of which are light and deteriorate less quickly than others.

The base or carrier oils should be carefully chosen as they contain certain benefits themselves, not least their content of iodine and vitamin E. They also act as a balancing and stabilising agent. The carrier oil should be pure and preferably cold pressed from the first pressing when it retains its vitamin content better. Later extractions use heat or solvent processes, which destroy the trace minerals and vitamins found in the oils.

Good base oils should have little or no smell of their own and should be penetrative.

The quantity of the carrier oil used will depend on the dryness / oilyness of the skin, the size of the client and the amount of bodily hair.

Grapeseed Oil – Vitis vinifera

The plant is a deciduous climbing vine. There are about 3000 different varieties of grape and most single grapes tend to only produce two seeds each.

The high-quality oil keeps well, is tasteless and almost colourless. It contains vitamins, minerals, and proteins and it does not contain cholesterol.

For massage it is less greasy, light and easily absorbed. Grapeseed oil has no contra-indications and therefore can be used on all ages and skin types.

Sweet Almond Oil – prunus amygdalis var dulcis

Cultivated for centuries and used in cookery throughout the world. The oil is best cold pressed but is more expensive that the solvent or heat extracted oil that is generally available.

This has usually lost a lot of the beneficial properties of the plant. For massage, always buy the best quality that you can afford.

It is probably the most popular oil for massage practitioners as it is light in colour and very oily. Chemically similar to peach, hazelnut and apricot kernels oils.

There are two types of almond tree – the bitter almond that produces white blossom and the sweet almond that produces pink blossom. We only use the sweet almond oil.

It is particularly good for dry itchy skin, baby's bottoms, eczema and sunburn.

It does not become rancid and it has very little smell. It contains glucosides, minerals, vitamins and is rich in protein.

Coconut Oil – Cocos nucifera

The fruit is a large drupe with a hard exterior, which contain milk and the solid nut from which the oil is extracted. At its best, it is cold pressed but it is often solvent extracted. It has a low viscosity and solidifies at 0°C. Rarely used in massage treatments but ideal for making locally applied mixes such as face creams or pain relieving balms.

Hypericum Oil – Hypericum perforatum

The common name is St John's Wort. When the buds are crushed 'hypericin' is released, staining the fingers blood red. It is in full flower on June 24th and takes its name from St John the Baptist because this is the St John's feast day.

In the Middle Ages it was hung around doorways to ward off evil spirits. The Knights of the Crusades used it to help heal sword wounds and modern evidence shows that it has bactericidal power. As a tea and nowadays a supplement it is recommended for depression. Samual Gray in 1818 recommends a tincture for 'maniacal and melancholic' illness and there is evidence of its use that dates back 2000 years.

Its properties are anti-inflammatory, antiseptic, analgesic, astringent diuretic, calming, and healing. It is said to be a natural antibiotic.

It will speed the healing of wounds, bruises, varicose veins, and mild burns. It is especially useful on sunburn, as it will help lower skin temperature.

Helps problems such as inflamed nerves as with sciatica, neuralgia, fibrositis and arthritis.

Never use undiluted for a full body massage. Use 4 mls of Hypericum added to a 12 mls of either Grapeseed or Almond for a full body massage. This will increase the beneficial quality of the treatment.

Sunflower Oil – Helianthus annus

Some organically cold pressed oil is available and this is light in texture and pleasant to use. This is sometimes used as a macerating medium for such plants as marigolds and violets. It contains vitamins A, B, D and E and several minerals. It is useful in the treatment of skin problems, bruises and ulcers. Cosmetically it has a soothing and moisturizing effect on the skin. Unfortunately most sunflower oil is solvent extracted and not really suitable for Aromatherapy.

Jojoba Oil – Simmondsia sinensis or Buxus sinensis

This oil is really a wax. It is not composed of triacylglycerols but a long chain of fatty acids. It has a long shelf life, as it does not oxidize. It will solidify if kept in the fridge.

It comes from the bean or seed of a perennial shrub that grows in desert terrain.

It has a long-standing use by the American Indians in Mexico and Arizona where the beans grow wild.

Jojoba is highly penetrative. Used as an addition to other base oils it helps skin and hair problems. Contains protein, minerals, has antibacterial qualities and a waxy substance that mimics collagen. It is a extremely good facial oil. Use for sunburn, psoriasis and acne or any congested skin condition.

Calendula Oil

This oil is extracted from the marigold flowers with the use of other vegetable oils. It has cosmetic uses and is often added to other base oils.

It is particularly useful for itching, menopausal / hormone related problems and skin complaints such as psoriasis, eczema, bruising, chapped skin, nappy rash, bed sores and broken veins.

It is a macerated product so it is worth remembering that if this is included in a blend, a certain amount of essential oils from the flower are already present in the oils.

Use up to 25% in your massage treatment.

PREGNANCY

Aromatherapy can be used safely and beneficially to maintain the general health of the expectant mother and to help minimise the various discomforts of pregnancy such as nausea, backache, swollen legs and ankles. Essential oils balance the body and a regular massage is beneficial on both a physical and emotional level.

Aromatherapy has a definite and beneficial role to play in 'natural' childbirth although it should not be considered to take the place of allopathic medicine. Although beneficial during pregnancy we must look very carefully at the oils that could possibly harm mother or foetus.

The following oils should **NOT** be used during the pregnancy at all mainly because of their Ketone and Phenol content and although none have been proved to be harmful (except in large doses) it is unwise to use any of the following oils or any oils that you are not completely familiar with:

Angelica, Aniseed, Basil, Camphor, Cinnamon, Clove, Fennel, Hyssop, Lemongrass, Myrrh, Nutmeg, Oreganum, Sage, Savory, Thyme, Tarragon, Pennyroyal, Wintergreen.

Oils that should be **AVOIDED** in the first 6 months:

Juniper, Lavendin, Marjoram, Cajuput, Caraway, Clary Sage, Rosemary, Cypress, Myrrh, Niaouli, True Melissa, And Pine.

The following oils **CAN BE SAFELY USED** during pregnancy (after the first 3 months):

Bergamot, Chamomiles, Frankincense, Grapefruit, Geranium, Lavender, Jasmine, Pine, Orange, And Ravensara.

These oils can be used safely during the whole pregnancy:

Cedarwood, Neroli, Eucalyptus R, Ginger, Tea Tree, Lemon, Sandalwood, Mandarin, Rose Otto, Petigrain, Ylang Ylang.

Essential oils do cross the placenta but have been filtered by the time they reach the foetus. The placenta is extremely selective and because they are natural molecules, the body knows how to deal with them.

The following recipes can be used safely after the first few months.

Morning Sickness

1 drop of peppermint in a glass of honeyed water first thing in the morning.

General Nausea

Use a burner with a mixture of **Eucalyptus** and **Lavender**. A lovely smell, relaxing, uplifting and antiseptic. Also try **Sweet Orange** and **Petigrain.**

Stretch Marks (prevention)

Mix 100 mls chosen carrier oil (almond, grapeseed) with 7 drops of each **Lavender, Mandarin** and **Frankincense** or **Neroli, Lavender** and **Chamomile**

Liberally apply to body, neck to knees daily.

Insomnia

Only use **Lavender** (angustifolia) 2 drops on a pillow at night.

Sandalwood and **Ylang Ylang** in a vaporiser in the bedroom before retiring can help too.

Varicose Veins

Use before rising in the morning the following mixture:

Mix 100mls oil or lotion with 7 drops of each **Cypress, Lemon** and **Lavender,** or 10 drops of each **Geranium** and **Cypress.**

Back Pain

Use any of the oils that are safe for pregnancy before 6 months. Use 5 drops of each **Rosemary** and **Lavender** in a warm bath, or the same mixed with 50 mls of carrier oil for massage after the first 6 months. Try **Roman Chamomile** and **Lavender** together too.

Constipation

Lotion with any of the **CITRUS** oils massaged into the lower abdomen.

Mood Changes

There are many conflicting emotions during pregnancy that are both confusing and upsetting for the mother. Essential oils are marvellous to help lift spirits. 10 drops of **Clary Sage** oil on a tissue tucked into the bra can keep moods at bay and help the mother remain cheerful and alert. **Geranium, Rose Otto, Neroli, Chamomile** and **Jasmine** are also good for balancing the emotions.

PREPARATION FOR LABOUR

Towards the end of pregnancy around the 8th month some of the previously forbidden oils are excellent.

Sage and Fennel strengthen the womb. **Cypress and Rosemary** will ease aching limbs.

During labour, make a treatment oil of **Rose Otto, Geranium and Clary Sage or Rosemary, Neroli and Frankincense** and use to massage the patients back, arms, hands and legs. Both mixes are wonderful for the nervous system and facilitate easy breathing. The calming effect increases the oxygen supply to the blood and brain and helps the woman avoid hyperventilation. They are also antiseptic and disinfectant.

For a foot massage use **Chamomile, Sandalwood and Mandarin** in a dilution of carrier oil to relax during the waiting period. **Ginger** if nauseous.

Try 1 or 2 drops of **Neroli, Peppermint, Basil** mixed together in a diffuser or vaporiser.

POST NATAL CARE

Cracked Nipple Oil

Use only pure **Almond or Calendula** oil.

Healing the Perineum

5 drops of **Cypress** and 5 drops of **Lavender** in the bath. Neroli is good too but best applied in a cream: 1-2 drops to 10mls cream.

To Promote Lactation

An ancient remedy for promoting lactation is to chew Fennel seeds and although it has not yet been established scientifically the use of the following oils can be tried **Fennel, Clary Sage, Lemongrass.**

Use a single oil 15 drops to 50 mls carrier oil and massage gently into the breast every day. Wash off thoroughly before feeding the baby.

To Stop Lactation

5 drops **Cypress,** 5 drops **Peppermint,** 5 drops **Lavender** with 50 mls carrier oil. Applied 3 or 4 times daily.

Haemorrhoids

6 to 8 drops of **Cypress** in the bath.

Post Natal Depression

The following oils strengthen the nervous system and lift depression:

Bergamot, Neroli, Clary Sage, Grapefruit, Geranium and Rose.

Try a mixture of **Rose, Bergamot and Clary Sage or Geranium, Neroli** and **Grapefruit.**

Mix together in a separate bottle and simply add a few drops of oil to a diffuser. Use the blend in the bath or mixed with a carrier oil for a massage.

Mastitis

Geranium, Lavender & Fennel. Mix with Calendula or Almond base oils and massaged into the breast 3 to 4 times a day. Other considerations – Diet, Underwear, Antiperspirant.

Essential Oils to Use After a Miscarriage

Choose a single oil or blend mix – **Rose Otto, Frankincense, Geranium, Grapefruit and Chamomile.**

INDIVIDUAL PRESCRIPTION

Now that you are familiar with the different uses and constituents of the forty essential oils and the base oils used in massage, you can start to consider how to construct an Individual Prescription.

Start by making a chart as shown on the following page for each individual system of the body – **Reproductive, Immune, Nervous, Genito-Urinary, Respiratory, Digestive, Head** and **Scalp, Circulatory, Endocrine, Skin,** and one for **Pregnancy** or any particular area that you work in.

List as shown the particular area of all the problems you come across in the first column under each of the systems and use the other three columns to donate which oils will treat those particular conditions. Study and read each oil profile, look for the uses described and fill in your charts as appropriate. Put the name of the oils in the column of notes that each belongs to.

This makes the decision about blending an **Individual Prescription** easy.

It is always important to do a detailed case study profile of each new client so that you are able to specifically treat the problems they present.

Include previous conditions, operations or treatments, medication, dietary habits, exercise, hobbies and family / genetic traits as well as the symptoms that they present before their treatment.

Leave a designated area on your health profile sheet to accommodate a set of cross-referencing charts.

Once you have a set of charts, cross-referencing is easy. Simply study your profiles and decide which of the client's problems are the most pressing. It is easiest to take three and cross-reference those.

See Case Studies.

SKELETAL AND MUSCULAR SYSTEM

TOP	MIDDLE	BASE
ACHES & PAINS		
Eucalyptus G	Lavender	Ginger
Clary Sage	Lavendin	Benzoin
Orange	Marjoram	Cedar
Thyme	Juniper Berry	Wood
Lemon Grass	Cypress	Neroli
Niaouli	Pine	
Orange	Ravensara	
Lemon	Chamomile	
Tea Tree	Black Pepper	

TOP	MIDDLE	BASE
ARTHRITIS / RHEUMATISM		
Lemon	Lavender	Ginger
Eucalyptus	Lavendin	Benzoin
Clary Sage	Marjoram	
Orange	Rosemary	
Thyme	Ravensara	
May Chang	Geranium	
	Black Pepper	
	Juniper	
	Pine	
	Cypress	

TOP	MIDDLE	BASE
STIFFNESS		
Lemon	Chamomile	Ginger
Niaouli	Lavender	Pine
Grapefruit	Lavendin	Benzoin
	Rosemary	
	Black Pepper	
	Marjoram	
	Pine	
	Fennel	

TOP	MIDDLE	BASE
CRAMP		
Basil Lemon Grass Bergamot	Marjoram Rosemary Peppermint Cypress	Ginger

TOP	MIDDLE	BASE
OSTEOPOROSIS		
Eucalyptus Lemon Grass Lemon	Lavender Rosemary	Benzoin Vetivert

TOP	MIDDLE	BASE
SCIATICA		
Thyme	Marjoram Black Pepper Ravensara	Ginger

TOP	MIDDLE	BASE
MUSCULAR PAIN / SPRAIN / SWELLING		
Eucalyptus G Clary Sage Grapefruit	Chamomile Lavender Marjoram Peppermint Rosemary Black Pepper	Rose Jasmine Benzoin Ginger

EXAMPLE OF A CASE STUDY

Jim – 55 years old. Contract engineer for 20 years. His general health is good but he has problems with his bowels and it has been diagnosed as IBS. He has had a lot of minor infections lately and feels a bit down in the dumps. Says he is always tired.

Likes a variety of food and at first glance his diet looks quite good but he eats a lot of red meat, too many carbohydrates and drinks excessively at weekends. His consumption of water is nil. He has a nagging shoulder and neck pain.

His job is not heavy work but he likes to get his hands dirty now and again with a bit of building work. His contract finishes in the next month and he is unsure what he will be doing next. For the first time in his life he doesn't have another job to go to and he is much more worried than he admits. He is a stone or so overweight but has recently started to play golf. He has come for a treatment because he isn't sleeping well and feels low.

First choice of oils would be immune boosting. It is obvious that he needs something to help his immune system as he has little energy and keeps getting minor infections. His digestive problems probably stem from his eating habits and lack of water. The second choice of oils would be for the IBS and constipation. The third choice would be for his neck and shoulder pain.

This is how your profile page will look. Immediately we can see the oils that will treat all of the three conditions:

Top notes: Tea Tree, Orange and Lemon

Middle notes: Lavender, Chamomile

Base notes: Ginger, Cedar Wood

Immune System			IBS			Muscular/Skeletal		
Top	**Mid**	**Base**	**Top**	**Mid**	**Base**	**Top**	**Mid**	**Base**
Berg	Geranium	Frank	Berg	Cham	Ginger	Euc G	Cham	Ginger
T.Tree	Lav	Rose	T.Tree	Lav	Rose	Orange	Lav	C.Wood
Lemon	Cham	Ginger	L. Grass	Jun	Neroli	Lem	Jun	Neroli
Bas	MarJ	Sand	Lemon	Pep	C.Wood	C.Sag	B.Pep	Benz
G.Fruit	Lavend	Benz	L. Grass	B.Pep	Neroli	L. Grass	Lavend	Cyp
Orange	Raven	.Wood	Orange	Fen	Mell	Niaouli	Marj	Pine
						T.Tree	Raven	

When you get used to blending you will easily pick those oils that blend well. In this case I would choose one from each of the different notes

So **Orange, Lavender and Ginger** would be my initial choice.

Depending on the activities after the treatment and the time of day should also be taken into consideration.

For a morning massage, I would choose **Lemon, Lavender and Chamomile.**

For an evening massage, I would probably blend **Chamomile, Ginger and Cedar wood.**

Now you have an INDIVIDUAL PRESCRIPTION for Jim.

He would be advised to drink more water, cut down on the red meat and carbs. Practice some gentle stretches for his neck and shoulders and to take time every day to eliminate properly at the same time every day.

Try the next three for yourselves:

Number 1. Linda – 28, 18-weeks pregnant with first baby
Subject is happy to be pregnant but experiencing lots of discomfort in her back, breasts and has mood swings. Finds she is easily irritated at the moment. Has indigestion most days.

She has been married for two years and her husband is away a lot. She is working in a busy estate agency and intends to carry on as long as possible.

She feels that her work is stressful, particularly as she does not get on well with her colleagues. Her general health is good but her diet is poor and she has always suffered with constipation and PMS.

She has a slight cough and complains of always having a sore throat. She smokes about 4 cigs daily and is trying really hard to cut them out altogether. She takes a multi vitamin pill daily.

She has come for a treatment mainly because her back is bothering her at the moment.

Work out an Individual Prescription for Linda and explain what advice you would give her.

Number 2. Maud – 80-year-old widow in an old peoples home

Is quite active and cheerful. Likes to read and watch TV. Plays bowls occasionally and still likes old time dancing when she gets the opportunity.

She has a long-term dry eczema which bother her quite a bit. She eats well and takes a tot of whiskey every night.

She gets very swollen ankles and has athlete's foot rather badly on one foot. Her blood pressure is slightly high, and she gets breathless easily.

She is also a moody person and gets easily irritated. Recently she has complained of a lot of neck pain, which often results in a headache.

Maud's family visits regularly and have noticed how bad tempered she is lately.

Work out an Individual Prescription for Maud and explain what advice you would give her.

Number 3. Jeffrey – 55-year-old company manager

Works in a large supply company and spends a lot of time away from home every week.

He stays in small hotels and pubs and usually works until 9pm so eats late and has a few drinks to unwind. He lives with his sister, as he is divorced.

He has come mainly because he finds it hard to relax and would like an evening massage so that he can get a good night's sleep. He has high blood pressure and gets breathless easily. He has type-2 diabetes and takes medication for both. He says he is careful about his diet since being diagnosed.

Work out an Individual Prescription for Jeffrey and explain what advice you would give him.

Later in this guide are the choices I would have made and the advice I would have given.

RECIPES

The following are a few example recipes that show just how versatile the oils that we have studied really are! The mixes are generally a Top, Middle and Base note, which gives a balanced treatment.

A=Application, **B**=Bath, **C**=Compress, **I**=Inhalation,**M**=Massage

ACNE: **Grapefruit/Lav/Patchouli. A, B, M.**
Other considerations – Diet, Stress, Age.

ASTHMA: **Basil/Marjoram/Frankincense. A, B, M.**
Other considerations – Diet, Stress, Chemicals

ARTHRITIS: **Eucalyptus R/Pine/Benzoin. A, B, C, M.**
Other considerations – Diet, Exercise, Warmth

BACK PAIN: **ClarySage/R-mary/Ginger. A, B, M.**
Other considerations – Posture, Exercise.

CELLULITE: **Grapefruit/JuniperBerry/Patchouli. A, B, M.**
Other considerations – Diet, Water, Skin Brushing.

COLD SORES: **Bergamot/Geranium/Patchouli.**   **A.**
Other considerations – General immune health.

CRAMP: **Basil/Lavender/Ginger. A, B, M.**

Other considerations – Exercise, Relaxation, Mineral deficiency.

CONSTIPATION: **Mandarin/BlackPepper/Patch. A, B, M.**

Other considerations – Diet, Exercise, Water intake, Habit

DEPRESSION: **May Chang/Geranium/Neroli. A, B, I, M.**

Other considerations – Lifestyle, Diet, Exercise / Relaxation, Vit Supplements.

ECZEMA: DRY: **Geranium, Chamomile.**

                     WET: **Juniper Berry, Lavender. A, B, M.**

Other considerations – Stress, Diet, Life-style, Sensitivities.

HANGOVER: **Grapefruit/MayChang/Rosemary. A, B, I, M.**

Other considerations – Dependency, Relaxation, Stress.

HEADACHE: **Lemon/R-mary/Peppermint. A, B, I, M.**

Other considerations – Spine, Exercise, Digestion, Diet, Fresh Air, Stress.

INSOMNIA: **Clary Sage/Lavender/Rose. A, B, I, M.**

Other considerations – Stress, Stimulants, Diet, Exercise, Fresh Air, Relaxation.

MENOPAUSE: Basil/Geranium/Ylang Ylang. A, B, I, M.

Other considerations – Diet, Exercise, Vitamin Supplements.

P.M.S: **ClarySage/Marjoram/Ginger. A, B, M.**

Other considerations – Diet, Exercise, Vitamin Supplements, Warmth

SINUS: **Tea Tree/Lavendin/Cedarwood. A, I, M.**

Other Considerations – Diet, Chemicals, Congested tears

VARICOSE VEINS: Lemon/ Rosemary/Patch. A, B, C.

Other Considerations – Diet, Exercise, Relaxation.

RESULTS OF CASE STUDY EXERCISE

CASE STUDY 1 – LINDA

The first column on our health profile will be Stress and Mood swings.

The second column will be for her Backache. (This is the reason for her appointment with you.)

The third column we will list the Digestive oils to help her Indigestion.

Because Linda is 18 weeks' pregnant, we will list only those oils we know to be safe.

Stress / Mood Swings			Backache			Indigestion		
Top	**Mid**	**Base**	**Top**	**Mid**	**Base**	**Top**	**Mid**	**Base**
Berg	Ger	Frank	Berg	Cham	Ginger	Lem	Lav	Ginger
T.Tree	Lav	Rose	T.Tree	Lav	Rose	Berg	Cham	Neroli
Lem	Cham	Ging	Orange	Raven	Neroli	G Fruit		
G.Fruit	Raven	Sand	Lemon		C.Wood	Orange		
Orange		C.Wood						

There are masses of choices here:

Firstly it's easy to see that the citrus oils would be both safe and beneficial so my initial choice.

Linda's *Individual prescription* would be **Bergamot / Chamomile / Ginger.**

If she has a day off and can relax but bearing in mind that she might be going to work later, then my choice would be **Lemon / Lavender / Chamomile**.

Base Oil: Grapeseed

Advice given: Obviously she must stop smoking! Eat plenty of nourishing food and increase her water intake. Do some basic stretches daily to help her backache. I would suggest that a mix to prevent stretch marks would be beneficial.

CASE STUDY: 2 MAUD 80 years old

Eczema/Athlete's foot			High Blood Pressure			Headaches/Neck Pain		
Top	**Mid**	**Base**	**Top**	**Mid**	**Base**	**Top**	**Mid**	**Base**
Berg	Ger	Patch	C.Sage	Marj	Ylang	Eur R	Cham	Neroli
Orange	Lav	Rose	May C	Lav	Rose	Bas	Lav	C.Wood
T.Tree	Cham	Benz	Lem	Jun	Neroli	Lem	Jun	
Niaouli	Jun	Neroli				L.Grass	R'mary	
P.Rosa		S.Wood				Niaouli	Marj	

A little more difficult as Maud is eighty and we do not want to use very strong oils on her.

Juniper comes up as a middle note but there at not three oils in the top notes. Top note **Niauoli** will treat eczema / athlete's foot and headaches. Base note **Neroli** treats all three problems so I would choose that.

Individual Prescription for Maud: **Niaouli/Juniper/Neroli.**

Base oil: Almond with 25% Calendula.

Advice given: I would like to see Maud soak her feet in a Tea Tree dilution to clear up the athlete's foot. A lotion for the eczema would perhaps stop her irritability (the body and mind are closely inter-related). Perhaps Orange, Geranium and Rose in a white lotion or calendula oils. There are many different oils that help skin condition.

CASE STUDY 3 – JEFFREY

Relaxation			Diabetes			High Blood Pressure		
Top	**Mid**	**Base**	**Top**	**Mid**	**Base**	**Top**	**Mid**	**Base**
Berg	Ger	Frank	C.Sage	Lav	Ginger	C.Sage	Marj	Ylang
Palma	Cham	Jas	Euc G	Jun	Rose	Lem	Lav	Rose
Bas	Lav	Rose	G Fruit	Ger	Neroli	May C	Jun	Neroli
Lem G	Mar	Ylang	Bas					
G.Fruit	Cyp	Benz						
Orange	Raven	Neroli						

Once again we don't have three top notes but **Grapefruit** treats the first two problems and **Clary Sage** the second two. Either will blend well with the others.

Middle notes **Lavender** is the only one that treats all
Base note **Neroli** is the other obvious choice.

Individual prescription for Jeffrey: **Grapefruit/Lavender/Neroli**
Clary Sage/Lavender/Neroli

Either mixes would be suitable for an evening massage but I would pick the mix with Clary Sage as I know this is extremely relaxing even though it is a top note.

Advice given: Increase water intake. Try to eat the evening meal a bit earlier and take a bit of time to do some regular exercise. Of course, I would recommend a regular massage treatment!

About the Author

In her working years, Joy Burnett was a practicing Aromatherapist, Reflexologist, and Holistic Healthcare Practitioner.

In 1990, she worked with AIDS patients for Cleveland Aids Support and wrote a clinical thesis on the immune system, some of which is published in Shirley Price's 'Aromatherapy for Health Professionals.'

In 1993, Joy opened her own school in North Yorkshire, The Rainbow Bridge School of Aromatherapy' accredited nationally by ISPA the International Society of Professional Aromatherapists and taught to a high level of expertise.

For over 11 years, Joy tutored and practiced her art there. Her students studied Aromatherapy for 14 months and were encouraged to extend their knowledge in other natural disciplines. Many became known in the North East as professional healthcare practitioners working alongside the NHS, supporting their work with children, cancer patients, in hospices, with pregnancy and the elderly, improving the relationship between modern and traditional medicine.

***

Now retired, Joy writes, directs amateur theatre, and enjoys travelling.

Having lived in Oman, Brunei, Abu Dhabi and Spain, she now lives in Northamptonshire, UK.

After joining a local writers group, Joy was inspired to start writing novels, the first of which is 'On the Loose', and she is already planning others. She is also the author of the short story collection 'All at Sea'.

***

Note from the Author

Thank you for purchasing 'Aromatherapy for Massage Practitioners'.

I hope you found it helpful and I would be very grateful if you would leave a review at your favourite online store and / or book-related website. Thank you.

If you would like a full set of charts to use for cross-referencing, please contact me and I will send you details of how to purchase them.

If you would like to know more about my writing, I would love to hear from you.

My email address is joyburnettwriter@yahoo.co.uk.